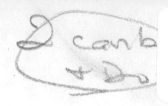

THE PATRIARCHAL VOICE

*Turn Your
Hidden Persuader
into a
Powerful Ally*

Mary King

Praise for The Patriarchal Voice

"In her recent book about female wine makers, <u>Crushed By Women</u>, Jeni Port remarks that for many women in the professional arena, "many of the battles of the past have been won." She goes on to explain that, in order to succeed, women should no longer feel the need to be 'one of the boys.' In fact, as more and more women break through into the top of their field, many professionals can at last look forward to simply being 'one of the gals.'

But, in <u>The Patriarchal Voice</u>, author and professional pharmacist, Mary King, reminds us that this is far from the case, particularly for those women who find themselves at the tips of the branches of feminist discussion. As a successful professional, and as an eager and actively aware participant in life, Mary has also had occasion to examine specific gender roles and their implications for the aspiring modern woman. Her book offers an instructive personal perspective on women's issues, particularly for those of us who have been left out of the dialogue. Indeed, <u>The Patriarchal Voice</u> offers a valuable new entry point into the conversation, invited and guided by the insightful personal extrapolations of a keen commentator.

Mary King's new book accompanies other recent publications such as The American Psychological Association's, <u>The Counselling Psychologist, Feminist Identity Development</u>; not to mention the impending return of Germaine Greer to our shores. We are *reminded that new perspectives are always instructive, and that vigorous dialogue concerning the status of women should continue into the next century. Discussion ensures that all women will become aware of the victories of the past and the challenges for the future."*

Anne Regan B.A., M.Ed.
Careers Consultant Regan Consulting Pty Ltd

"Mary King's <u>The Patriarchal Voice</u> *has an important and timely healing message for us all, both women and men. Her wisdom and insight into the deeply held beliefs that underpin our actions can help us break free from archaic and damaging behaviour patterns. This book is empowering for both sexes, and will inspire many people to make important changes in their lives."*

Michelle Michie
Managing Director Nicholson Media Group

"Mary King's <u>The Patriarchal Voice</u> *is not about 'men versus women', although as I read it there were times when I thought it was! It is about the dynamic relationship between the masculine and feminine aspects within all people. As such, it is an important contribution to each of us understanding ourselves at a deeper level."*

Ian McDonald
Corporate Development Consultant

"The Patriarchal Voice will definitely be on my 'to buy' list for all the women in my life that I care about. I found myself in so many of the pages and as a practising psychotherapist I know how important it is to 'name' what is happening for us on an unconscious level before we tackle it. We all, men and women, will thank Mary King for writing for us a book that will surely change, for the better, the lives of all who read it."

Margaret Seedsman
Psychotherapist

"It is surprising how we travel through life not being aware of the Patriarchal Voice which is firmly lodged within our subconscious minds. The Patriarchal Voice should be read by ALL women regardless of age, profession and marital status. Mary King has written this book in a conversational, easy-to-read and thought provoking manner. She clearly communicates how we can recognise the Patriarchal Voice and change our lives."

Kay Watts AIMS, BA(Soc Sc), MA(Mgmt)
National Sales Manager Australian Biotechnology News

"The Patriarchal Voice is inspiring reading. Poignant reality brings home truths alive, offering logical examples of subliminal conditioning."

Christine Griffiths
Managing Director Ivy Industries

"Mary King has done it again; she has taken the risk of baring much of her soul to help her readers gain insights into their often unconscious patterns of behaviour. I admire her courage in doing so. I gained valuable perspectives from <u>The Patriarchal Voice</u>, and recommend it to both men and women. These perspectives help in developing self-awareness, which I believe is the key to living the conscious life that Socrates recommended so long ago!"

Charles Kovess LL.B. (Hons), LL.M., CSP
Author of best-selling
<u>Passionate People Produce</u> and <u>Passionate Performance</u>

"I totally loved <u>The Patriarchal Voice</u>! Beautifully written and simply explained. It brought to consciousness my inner voice therefore allowing me more choice in my everyday life. Mary King has a special way with words. I totally support her quest for bringing completion to the women's movement to achieve harmony and equality for all."

Anna Hamilton
Professional Member Tarot Guild of Australia
and The Australian Psychics Association,
Former President Global Energy Network Institute
(GENI) Foundation Ltd

"Mary King offers simple truth which gives some direction towards healing our hearts. To empower our inner voice we need to hear the loving voice of the feminine power."

Dr Janet Hall, Psychologist, Sex Therapist, TV Personality and Author of several books including Boss Of The Bladder, Toddler Taming, Fight-Free Families and Confident Kids

"The Patriarchal Voice is a personal account of Mary King's journey of discovery of the effects on her of her Patriarchal Voice, bringing it to consciousness, and forming a healing relationship with it."

Pam Salmon
Grad. Dip. Counselling, Cert. Mediation Counselling, Member Victorian Parole Board, Former Senior Manager Dept. Human Services

" ... Mary King gets you thinking. You may not agree with everything she says but she has the courage to say what she thinks. If you want your thinking provoked read The Patriarchal Voice."

Kevin Bolt
MD Operation Transformation Pty Ltd

"Over the years I have witnessed much human suffering. When the soul has been repressed from early childhood by the Patriarchal Voice, more often than not the child continues to abuse himself or herself by giving voice to the critic it has become used to. I sincerely hope that understanding and harnessing this Patriarchal Voice enables future generations to go for their dreams and look forward to loving and fulfilling lives. I am honoured to be involved in such a worthwhile and important project, and hope you enjoy <u>The Patriarchal Voice</u> as much as I have."

Susan Barton Founder The Lighthouse Foundation
Tattersall's Award for Enterprise and Achievement 1994
The Australian Humanitarian Award for Education 1998
NAB Community Link Award for Community Services 1999
Victoria Day Award for Community and Public Service 2000
Author with Katherine Ingram
<u>Build Your Teenager's Self Esteem</u>

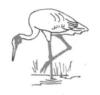

Published by Brolga Publishing Pty Ltd
P.O. Box 959, Ringwood,
Victoria, 3134, Australia

National Library of Australia
Cataloguing-in-Publication entry
King, Mary
The Patriarchal Voice

ISBN 0-9096088-5-7

Cover Design: Trish Hart   Artwork By: Dympna Lodge
Typset By: Wendy Aird   Edited By :   Pauline Luke

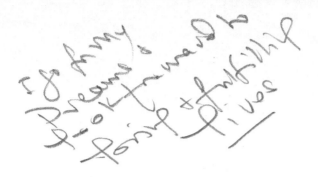

The Patriarchal Voice is the embodied voice of the patriarchy passed from generation to generation for centuries. Operating in the mind it expresses the ideas and rules of the dominant philosophy of the patriarchal system. Put simply, *if it is feminine it is inferior.*

In men its effect is to restrict their ability to be open to their emotions and their vulnerability. In women it hinders their progress, inhibits their ability to speak and makes them doubt not only themselves, but also other women.

By learning to recognise this voice within ourselves both men and women can evaluate its limiting beliefs. Then we have a chance to change our responses so that we empower ourselves and our relationships.

For
my parents
Jack and Ann McDonnell

Self Independent
+
Assured
+

Nice!
Comfort +
Reasonant

Acknowledgments

When I decided to delve into my Patriarchal Voice I became more aware of the same voice in those around me. I thank all those people who gave me material that I used in the book. Many of those who know me may find a little of our experience in the following pages. I'm grateful to each person who either gave me a situation so I could learn, or shared their experience with me.

Thanks to my editor Pauline Luke, who read the first draft and has guided me through updates. I sincerely appreciate her willingness to grasp a reasonably challenging topic and make helpful suggestions. She has been invaluable to me.

I would especially like to thank Robin Gale-Baker for her assistance and support with the writing of this book. When I was blocked Robin was able to lead me to clarity so I could complete the work. Robin has an excellent understanding of the Patriarchal Voice. I greatly appreciate her input.

To Sidra Stone, who wrote about the inner patriarch in her book <u>The Shadow King</u>, thank you so much for helping me learn more about my Patriarchal Voice and facilitating me in separating it from my other voices. To Hal Stone, thank you for gently making me aware how I let my Patriarchal Voice do the talking.

Thank you to my family - my grown children and partners, my brothers, sisters and sisters by marriage for your on-going support. Thanks especially to John and Noel for letting me use the beach house to write.

Thanks to my friend Dympna Lodge for her artwork.

Thanks to Brolga Publishing, Wendy Aird, Trish Hart, and Mark Zocchi for making it so easy to excellently publish a book.

Contents

Introduction

I wrote this book from my own experience, of discovering my Patriarchal Voice, bringing it to consciousness, making it my friend and healing my relationship with it. This awareness is the result of a journey spanning many years towards my goal for a close, personal, fulfilling and on-going relationship with a man.

Without this personal discovery it is my belief I would not be able to sustain a lasting partnership. My Patriarchal Voice was in charge in that area of my life and I was a victim under its control. I was vaguely aware of its presence but I had no idea of the extent of its influence. I discovered it annihilated my ability to believe in myself.

For six thousand years the dominant philosophy of our society has been patriarchal (men are superior to women). The Patriarchal Voice has repeated patriarchal ideas inside the heads of women and men. We may not recognise that we have responded so faithfully to these subtle persuasions.

Patriarchal society has worked. Women and men knew their roles and worked together. It is only in relatively recent years that the women's movement and other anti-discrimination causes have brought heightened attention to inequalities existing among our people.

As you read on you may feel that I'm in judgement of the way it has been. I am not. We are all, both women and men, products and victims of patriarchal society. I love men and I love women. I believe they are meant to compliment and support each other. I simply want to do what I can to assist in the movement towards respect for all.

The external world reflects our internal world. Much has been done to make changes in the outer world. *This book is about changing our inner world.*

We may not realise we are being controlled from inside ourselves because that's the paradigm in which we live. Like a goldfish in a bowl sees only through its environment, we are immersed in patriarchal thinking. If we're not aware we may not realise how we are being affected.

My Patriarchal Voice seemed to get stronger as time passed. Because of the indignities I had suffered in my life it determined to protect me as only it knew how. The Patriarchal Voice was inside my head and I responded to its edicts in matters of self-esteem, unaware I was being influenced to such an extent.

My Patriarchal Voice was like a killer locked in a room in my psyche. It rid my life of potential male partners because it believed I was not good enough for them. I was a woman and as such I deserved neither liking nor approval.

It affected my vision so that I couldn't observe men as they really were. Either I saw them through rose coloured glasses and glossed over their defects or I looked through grey tinted glasses that caused me to emphasise their faults. It influenced my thinking, my feelings and my behaviour. In other words it acted as a filter of which I was unaware. All my experiences came through this filter. My reality was censored and controlled.

I know I'm not alone in this. I've listened to many single female friends and it is obvious to me they will not be able to sustain a relationship, unless they become aware, as I did, or at least make some internal changes. Even though they would like a partnership, and they are desirable people, there is a force at work that is powerful and beyond their immediate awareness.

In much the same way the Patriarchal Voice affects men by giving them unrealistic expectations and understandings of women, and limiting their ability to recognise and express their feelings.

Because the Patriarchal Voice speaks from the shadow of our psyche, it is not obvious to most of us the degree to which our lives are so strongly affected. We are not conscious this powerful force is directing our thoughts and actions. Some people display an obvious Patriarchal Voice, for example a man or woman who clearly upholds the status quo of patriarchal society in which women are inferior to men. In others it operates on an inner level and is almost impossible to hear in their everyday lives and yet the effect is experienced as not only a belittling but also a restriction of the feminine.

My reason for writing is to bring to consciousness a voice most of us, both male and female, are not aware of but will surely recognise. Although we are unaware it is happening this voice is operating in our mind and strongly affects our lives. This book is about making us conscious of some of our beliefs so that we may make changes in our inner world if we choose.

There are many advantages of using the Patriarchal Voice appropriately. These include access to clarity of thought, order, rules for guidance, some control over the situation, protection, a cool head, boundaries, limits, strength, courage, intellect, reason, armour, discipline, decisions, stability, ability to lead, dominion, non-dependence and good financial principles.

I trust that as you follow my journey you also discover the role of the Patriarchal Voice in your own life and learn to hear the competing and attacking thoughts that undermine your sense of self and entitlement.

1

Changes

"I see my patterns, and I choose to make changes."
Louise L. Hay <u>You Can Heal Your Life</u>

It was a restaurant party with dancing to music from a live band. I was sitting next to a man I had met before. Our conversation was lively and interesting. He asked me to dance. I love dancing and to my delight I found he was an excellent dancer and a masterful director.

That night I danced as never before. This man led and I followed. Other dancers watched as we moved together as one. He twirled me round and bent me back. I placed my trust in his direction and found myself supported. At one stage my feet even left the floor and I found myself lying on my back strongly held up on his bent knee. Because I was physically fit, I easily adapted to the strenuous pace demanded by his guidance. We danced together in superb rhythm and tempo.

Suddenly, as part of the dance, and in perfect timing, movement and cadence, he whacked me on the backside, causing me to cry out in shock and pain.

I was totally taken aback. I noticed myself express surprise and I watched myself keep on dancing. I was reminded of bondage. Why did I not immediately stop the dance? I felt abused and yet I did nothing to protest against the treatment I had received.

Later when I reflected on this experience I understood such incidents to be fairly common. Women suffer humiliation at the hands of men and they don't say anything about it or even prevent it from happening again. I believe it was my internalised Patriarchal Voice that prevented me from objecting publicly to the treatment I was subject to. I had not consciously given this man permission to hit me and I said and did nothing to prevent him from doing it again. A part of me (my Patriarchal Voice) decreed nothing untoward had happened and convinced me that all was well. I pondered the question, if a man found himself in a similar situation would he have retaliated?

As I thought about this incident I realised that men invade women's personal space when they touch them. A man pursuing a woman may intrude on her space and often she allows it, even though she may not welcome it. I have often found myself in the position of having a man move in on me. I have many times not been able to keep a distance between us. My Patriarchal Voice kept me silent.

Shortly after this experience I returned to the seaside to begin writing this book. Two years had passed since my last visit. I was astonished to see the changes to the coast. The ocean had encroached on the shore and was claiming the sand dunes and eroding the porous red rock. There was little beach left between me and the rushing water. I felt fearful as I pondered where to walk. I recalled my daughter, an environmental manager, telling me years earlier, "The coast doesn't care." It is we, the people, who care that change is happening. Change is inevitable. Nothing is as constant as change.

Because of the efforts of the women's movement in attempting to change the status of women and raise their profile, many men and women have responded and heeded the call. There have been many changes in society. Old movies remind us how it was for women just a few decades ago. When we are reminded how it was in the past we are often surprised. When we are part of a situation we can't always see what is happening in the bigger picture. When we look back we see that many women led lives that were difficult with much hardship compared with the relative comfort available in the First World today.

Many women lead lives that are less demanding physically today. Many have their own money, more freedom and a greater chance to be heard. Women have made great strides forward. The dreams of many include high aspirations such as achieving top positions in politics, business and corporations and living lives of choice regarding partners, children and marriage. They believe their goals are achievable and many feel hopeful. However, the reality may not be as promising as it seems. In spite of the advances most women still find themselves restrained.

Men have heard the voices of the feminists, many have realised the indignities suffered by women, seen the unequal treatment of men and women. Many men acknowledge that what happens for women is not 'right'. Some men are affected, some understand, others just don't want to know.

In the past the patriarchy often ruled with an iron fist. Many women felt rebellious at the rules and restrictions that seemed to stifle and choke. However, changes are happening. The pendulum is swinging the other way as society adapts to ideas of women's rights. Some advances are apparent but now many women find themselves isolated and alone as they battle to raise a family single-handed.

Similarly, men are struggling. Isolation is not a new experience for men - they intimately understand the feeling. The problem for many men today is that they feel lost. Many responded to the women's movement by respecting the female condition and understanding their plight. They became aware all was not well with women and some felt distress. Because the rules are changing many men are no longer sure of their direction. A few years ago the patriarchy had clear guidelines. Men raising a family today don't always know what is expected of them. In the past man was acknowledged as leader of the family and he gave the orders. With the upsurgeance in the women's movement many men are questioning their role and how they might best serve the family. Some men have disowned their Patriarchal Voice, many have become indecisive and lacking a clear direction.

A man disowns his Patriarchal Voice by suppressing it. He fears the ideas of the patriarchy and may abandon his ability to lead and direct. He may appear 'weak' when compared to a man who is strongly patriarchal. Even though he may not act from a patriarchal position, internally he may still be 'beaten up' by the Patriarchal Voice in his head that tells him he is 'weak'.

The Patriarchal Voice makes women put aside their own ideas, desires and wishes in favour of those of men in their lives. It makes them unsure of themselves. There was a time in my life when I realised I had no idea what I liked and what I wanted to do. As I grew up I believed I was part of a family and must obey the rules. My family was, like most families, led by a patriarch. The rules to be followed came mostly from the patriarchal society. I aligned my inclinations to those of the patriarchal family.

I didn't know what music, colours, perfume or clothes I liked. I didn't know what career I would prefer. I found myself unable to choose a restaurant. I would defer to others wishes and leave them with the choice. I could not confidently decide.

If I had a preference I would not have confidence to stay with my choice because my thoughts would have been undermined by the powerful voice in my head. It was easier to let others make decisions. I was being controlled unconsciously by an invisible, irresistible force.

Why did I, as a woman, need to be controlled? Why was the Patriarchal Voice so powerful in my psyche?

In The Whole Woman Germaine Greer says sociologists tell us patriarchal systems of men controlling women originated so men could be sure they really were the father of their offspring. Previously the basic family was mother, maternal grandmother, aunts and children. Male sexual partners came and went. The stable adult male was the mother's brother. About 5000 years ago matrilocal civilisations ruled in Europe; the most stable and loving societies known. They were invaded by patriarchal Indo-Aryan warriors who realised that women held high esteem because of their unique ability to bring new life into the world and represented a threat to their dominator style of leadership. Women had the power to make men desire them and they had to be controlled, hidden, dominated and their social status reduced from equal to that of property.

The dominators looked at the women's menstrual blood, which had been a sacred substance to sprinkle on fields or use in fertility ceremonies for tens of thousands of years, and called it 'unclean'. They looked at the pain some women experienced in childbirth and proclaimed that their god said it was punishment for their wickedness. When crops failed and natural disasters occurred it was the fault of women and their witching ways.

The voice of the outer patriarchy, who don't want women's influence to be too compelling, became internalised. The Patriarchal Voice is the result of centuries of conditioning. Because the indoctrination is so powerful and insidious it goes on unconsciously, still directing internally. The Patriarchal Voice doesn't want a woman to get too powerful so it instructs her to limit herself. This voice passes from generation to generation through women. Women help maintain the patriarchal system. They do it unconsciously through the Patriarchal Voice that operates below their conscious awareness. Marion Woodman in <u>The Ravaged Bridegroom</u> writes: "The sons and daughters of the patriarchy are, in fact, motherbound."

This voice speaks inside the heads of men and women throughout the world. It is the voice of the ancient patriarchy embedded in our consciousness and passed on through generations. As you read some of its pronouncements you may recognise you've heard them before.

It says:
"Women doctors are not as good as men doctors."
" A woman dentist isn't strong enough to pull teeth."
"She'll never make it. She's a woman."
"It doesn't matter what course she gets in to. She'll only be there for a short period and then she'll get married and have children."
"Women should speak after men."
"Professional women don't stay in the work force for long. It's a waste."
"A woman's place is in the home."
"The man pays."

"A woman should wait for a man to open the door."
"A woman without a man is not a real woman."
"What's wrong with her? Nothing that a good f...
wouldn't fix."
"Women can't read maps."
"A good job for a woman is to be a teacher, a nurse or
help people."
"In tennis a man should serve first. It's a sign of
weakness to let the woman serve first."
"Women should be on a pedestal."
"Women's periods. A good excuse to take days off work"
"Girl!"

Women are judged, limited and trivialised by the patriarchy. The Patriarchal Voice takes these declarations and repeats them. The voice operates in their heads. It gets mixed up with their other voices and they cannot distinguish that they are being trivialised and restricted.

In the past women needed to heed the direction of their Patriarchal Voice so they would be safe. In today's changing times women generally have more financial independence (although still not, on average, as much as men) and more freedom to make choices. The reality is that women are still held back, by both the inner and outer patriarchy, and it is the purpose of this book to bring to awareness these distinctions so that the changes, begun by the feminists, can continue to full manifestation.

In the first part of the book we will look at how the Patriarchal Voice became so effective, then we will discover some of its beliefs and rules and finally we will see what can be done to bring balance in our inner world so that the outer world reflects these changes.

2

The Patriarchy in Australia

"If we cannot reflect on and learn from the past and learn from our mistakes how can we move into the future?"

President of the Museum Board,
Professor David Penington

The first boat load of women who came to Australia from England arrived in Botany Bay in the 1800's. The women were for the use of men living in the colonies. These men were rough and tough and starved of the company of women. They swooped on the women and used them, as wives, as cooks and house-keepers. The women were treated as possessions.

I've heard it said the women of Australia today have a memory in their cells and psyche of the treatment these pioneer women received at the hands of the early settlers and convicts. Australian women are still reacting to experiences of their predecessors.

Different treatment has been afforded men and women in Australian history. A century ago as the men fought for a federation the women were also fighting for the same thing.

Louisa Lawson holds a special place in Australian letters, yet her name is little known. Throughout the 1890's she was the editor and chief financial backer of a radical magazine for women, the first of its kind in this country. The magazine was staffed entirely by females - writers, editors, even printers. But occasionally, Louisa Lawson allowed her son Henry to contribute.

Henry Lawson has risen to almost universal recognition as Australia's premier bush poet while his mother - who spent the last six months of her life in an asylum and was buried in 1920 a pauper - languishes in obscurity. Much the same could be said for the women who helped give birth to this nation. We've grown used to hearing the phrase 'the founding fathers' of Federation, but what about 'the founding mothers'?

 While women were overlooked, men's poor behaviour was considered acceptable. An article by Amanda Dunn in The Age April 29, 2001 is headed: 'The sins of Federation's fathers. The fathers of the nation were not all above the baser urges. Horsewhipping, duelling, womanising, sex and the older man. Welcome to the untold story of Australian Federation.'

According to Helen Irving, Federation and constitutional historian at Sydney's University of Technology, some of the key figures of Federation led personal lives that ranged from the colourful to the downright scandalous.

Similarly, in horse racing different standards applied for men and women. A thick white line wound its way through Flemington Racecourse for 40 years. It marked out a barrier to prevent women betting at the same enclosures as men and drinking in their bars, and was a symbolic reminder that, as Victoria Racing Club chairman L.K.S. MacKinnon declared, after Precocious (a horse owned and trained by a young woman) won the 1932 Grand National Steeplechase: "Horse training is not suitable for women. The engagement of jockeys and other duties connected with training are essentially jobs for men - simply it is not thought to be a woman's sphere." The trainer 22 year old Dorothy Shiel, was not allowed into the mounting yard to accept the trophy.

After his death, Bill Smith - a successful Queensland jockey in the early 1900s who lived in seclusion, never married and never donned his silks in the jockeys' room - was found to be a woman, Wilhelmina Smith. Posing as a man she rode unobtrusively through the prejudices that prevented women from racing horses.

Sidra Stone Ph.D., author of <u>The Shadow King</u>, was the first person to recognise and name the inner patriarch. Subsequently on trips to Australia she observed, even in the 1990's, that their Patriarchal Voices (inner and outer) are responsible for the women and men of Australia not liking each other. Her experience came from Voice Dialogue sessions with many Australians (see Chapter 15 for an explanation of Voice Dialogue.) I talked with Sidra about men and women and relationships in Australia. She said she believes this mutual dislike is a reason for dissatisfaction in relationships in this new century. I highly recommend reading Sidra Stone's book <u>The Shadow King</u> for a rich and full explanation of the inner patriarch and the many and varied expressions of the Patriarchal Voice.

The Patriarchal Voice is very persuasive. Because it undermines women, devalues their abilities and contributions, men don't fully appreciate women - and neither do women. In Australia the Patriarchal Voice has an extra edge because of the culture of 'cutting down tall poppies'.

The 'tall poppy syndrome' is supported by the Patriarchal Voice. I listened the other day to a woman speaking with dislike about an Australian actor who has succeeded in Los Angeles. Portia de Rossi (a pseudonym) appears weekly in the comedy series Ally McBeal. This woman spoke scornfully (from her Patriarchal Voice) of Portia's change of name, her false hair and her 'fake' appearance. The rest of the women (including me) said nothing. This woman could have been speaking from a voice that believed that 'natural' is best. The tone and vibration with which she made the comments alerted me that it was, in fact, her Patriarchal Voice.

In women the Patriarchal Voice operates from the shadows undermining their belief in their own knowledge. Perhaps this is a clue to why most women who experience rape say nothing. Who would believe them? This tendency is deeply ingrained. Some women only admit to being raped many years after the event. I spoke to two women friends who told of being raped, one by her ex-husband and the other when she was a student at University. When the latter accused her aggressor she was dismissed as having led him on. The patriarchy uses its force and power to negate women and what they do, and to acknowledge men and men's achievements.

The Patriarchal Voice restricts women's speech. It believes women are in danger if they speak out against men. Men are strong and able to retaliate. Men don't give in easily. They can fight on to victory. That is why most women don't speak out when confronted with misjudgments and abuse. Their Patriarchal Voice (inner) colludes with the outer patriarchy and recommends silence.

Recently I stood up for myself against a man's criticism. I felt the criticism was unjust and uncalled for. I held my ground. He persisted till finally I was in tears. I felt surprised and unprepared for his attack on me. I was so upset I cried for a couple of hours. Now, I sense my Patriarchal Voice is guarding to make sure something similar does not happen again. My Patriarchal Voice thought it unwise that I stand up to this man. At the time I chose not to heed the warning. Sometimes we need to take risks for a higher purpose.

3
How the Patriarchal Voice
Promotes Inequality

"Men get something from marriage that women never do. They get wives."

Susan Maushart Wifework

While we may think that a husband and a wife have equality the reality may be different. The Oxford English Dictionary defines Wife as - a woman; formerly in general sense, in later use restricted to a woman of humble rank or 'of low employment'. One of the definitions in the Concise Oxford Dictionary defines in part Wife as - old and rustic or uneducated woman.

For six thousand years the patriarchy has ruled. The Patriarchal Voice carries on the tradition inside our heads. It has become deeply embedded in our psyches, almost cellular. The women's movement and society, influencing government to introduce laws, have endeavoured to change the patriarchy. Beginning with the suffragettes claiming the right to vote, strides have been taken to change the status of women to one of equality with men, from equal pay to anti-discrimination laws protecting women's rights.

In spite of progress true liberation for women is still a fantasy. Germaine Greer writes in The Whole Woman, "It's time to get angry again."

Why are women the majority in the world's destitute? Why are they still disadvantaged? Why are they still victims to men? Why do they not hold equal or at least a third of senior management positions in corporations? Why are they still underlings?

The Patriarchal Voice sees men as better, more interesting, more valuable and worth more than women. It trivialises what women do and belittles women's value. This voice is unconscious in the heads of many men and women.

Society commonly uses derogatory words for women and their work. As a pharmacist I work with mainly female staff called 'girls' or, sometimes, 'chickadees'. Women working in supermarkets are often referred to as 'check-out chicks'.

Despite the fanfare about equal opportunity and women-friendly workplaces, corporate Australia still has a long way to go when it comes to including females among the senior ranks. A recent study by Alison Sheridan, a senior lecturer in the school of marketing and management at the University of New England, found that women occupied little more than 3.4 per cent of board seats on publicly listed Australian companies.

One reason for the lack of advancement of women to senior management positions in corporations may be that men usually recommend other men from their 'old boy' network of friends and associates. Another may be that women tend not to support or promote other women at work. Both reasons can be attributed to the Patriarchal Voices (inner and outer) of these men and women. The Patriarchal Voice says generally women are inferior to men. Simone de Beauvoir comments in The Second Sex, *"We must be careful to note that the presence of a woman chief or queen at the head of the tribe by no means signifies that women are sovereign therein: the ascension to the throne of Catherine the Great in no way modified the lot of the Russian peasant woman."*

If men and women work together in equal positions there is still an expectation that the woman is responsible for the emotional atmosphere in the environment. The Patriarchal Voice in both men and women expects that she will take responsibility for creating and maintaining a pleasant climate. In the woman the Patriarchal Voice could say: "It's up to you to keep the staff, the bosses and the customers happy." In the man it could say something like: "You've got better things to do than worrying about how people feel. Let the girls take care of that."

Different Standards for Men and Women

Patriarchal society has much to answer. Different standards apply for men and women. A new analysis by University of Melbourne's Susan Donath researching how men and women spend their first hour after arriving home from work found, "on arriving home, men's most common activity is eating and drinking, while women's most common activity is food and drink preparation."

These findings are supported by a British survey which showed working mothers feel overworked, underpaid and at breaking point from stress. Lack of support from both their managers and their spouses means most working mothers think they are emotionally damaging their children and putting their own health at risk. The survey of 5000 women was for Top Sante magazine. The Patriarchal Voices of the women remind them they are responsible for caring for the family emotionally and physically and the pressure builds as they take on tasks at home and work.

Fewer than one in three people given Australia's highest awards are women. Victorian Women's Trust executive director, Mary Crooks, said the Order of Australia award list reflected a general undervaluing of women's achievements. Ms Crooks said women are less likely to promote themselves. Women put the "cement into the social system", but their efforts went unnoticed and unpaid. "I'd be bold enough to say a lot of women's achievements are, on similar economic and social terms, more significant than men's," she said.

A Reason Why Women are Still Disadvantaged

The Patriarchal Voice restricts and limits women as part of a normal course of events making them feel uncomfortable. The examples just mentioned illustrate results that still occur in the world of business. In spite of advances and changes it is the inner world that is still limiting women beyond their conscious understanding. The following is a personal example that may show how women allow themselves to be restricted.

Playing golf has usually been demanding for me. Hitting a small ball a long distance down a fairway, approaching the green, and putting the ball into a hole creates many challenges. The game becomes even more stressful as my Patriarchal Voice reminds me of the advance of the people behind and tells me I will hinder their passage of play. With this constant nagging I waste no time in approaching my ball, choosing the appropriate club, swinging it without delay to send my ball on its way, often with less than best application.

One day I became aware just how influenced I was by this voice. A woman friend and I were joined by a man who had been playing alone and we continued as a threesome. I soon discovered he prided himself on being a good pupil of his dad who was a prize-winning golfer. This day he was practising for an impending match with his father. I watched in amazement as he addressed his ball, got down on his haunches to examine the lie, stood back to see where to aim, puzzled over which club to use, took a couple of practice swings and finally hit the ball. In other words *he held his space.* Magically the people behind us no longer seemed to be a pressure, my inner patriarch relaxed and I enjoyed my golf.

I became aware that this golfer and I had different inner dialogues. He was not at the mercy of his Patriarchal Voice as I was. Possibly he was a victim of his inner critic, but that's another story. For more information on other voices read my book The Intuitive Voice.

Speaking in Public

Similarly, because of their Patriarchal Voices, women are challenged more than men when speaking publicly. My Patriarchal Voice makes me obey the rules regarding the time allotted for me to speak.

I gave a speech at my daughter's wedding. I knew I was pushing some patriarchal boundaries when I chose to speak and the Patriarchal Voices of the family members insisted I limit the duration. My ex-husband kindly shared his allocation as I had something important to say. I talked about my daughter's younger days giving one example demonstrating her delightful character and I welcomed her husband to the family. I only spoke for five minutes as I was conscious (thanks to my Patriarchal Voice) of limiting the content and editing excess words. I was amazed when a speaker from the other family spoke at length. He used the opportunity to freely say what he wanted.

I believe the Patriarchal Voice is a major factor that prevents many women from speaking in public.

My Patriarchal Voice insists I limit myself when telling a joke. The result is I totally forget the content. Therefore,

I rarely tell jokes. My Patriarchal Voice reiterates: "Women shouldn't tell jokes. It's okay for men." If I do attempt to tell a joke I nervously stumble through it, usually forgetting a vital piece of information, and the result is generally not amusing.

At the 2000 Academy Awards Hilary Swank accepted an Oscar for best actress for her starring role in <u>Boy's Don't Cry</u> in which she played a girl masquerading as a boy. She was determined not to forget to thank anyone and wrote names on paper. "I knew I couldn't forget anyone," she said, apologetically. After speaking quickly for two minutes she said, "I'm almost done, I promise," no doubt at the prompting of her Patriarchal Voice. She concluded her two and a half minute speech by saying: "I pray for the day when we accept our differences, but celebrate our diversity." Amen to that.

At the same award presentation Gwyneth Paltrow introduced the candidates for the best actor. She won the award in 1999 for best actress and, referring to her acceptance speech, commented: "You probably remember how wimpy I was too." (It seems her inner critic and her Patriarchal Voice had their way with her!)

Kevin Spacey accepted the award for best actor for the 2000 awards. Although "stunned and speechless" he managed to speak with emotion for three and a half minutes. His Patriarchal Voice allowed him to be who he was (a man) and hold his space.

Women's Sexuality

Patriarchal energy within is entrenched. Even if we are not conscious of the voice speaking in our minds we can feel the judgement of the inner patriarch.

For example, the patriarch within keeps women's sexuality contained. We can feel his disapproval if we wear something suggestive. This attitude probably came from our relationships with our fathers. We were not able to seduce our fathers so we had to squash our sexuality. Once, when I was married, I attempted to seduce my husband and wore a sexy black lace bra that pushed up my breasts. He was unimpressed and I felt rebuffed. My Patriarchal Voice made sure I didn't repeat that behaviour.

The Patriarchal Voice restrains women's sexuality. He doesn't like it. He makes sure they don't display it. Women are sexual beings whose sexuality is curtailed by the Patriarchal Voice. He can label us 'cheap' if we show too much cleavage or leg, or if we act in an overtly sexual way.

My Patriarchal Voice disapproved of the front cover of a magazine showing a picture of a woman, her legs spreadeagled and her crotch openly displayed. At its urging I noticed myself feeling judgemental.

If a woman displays or flaunts her sexuality she is labelled unpleasant names that belittle. Similarly, in medieval times the patriarchy hated women and labelled them 'witches'. The reciprocal title for men 'wizard' does not have the same negative connotations. If a man and woman have intercourse on 'a one night stand' the woman is in danger of 'losing her good name', whereas a man is excused as 'sowing wild oats'. He cannot 'sow wild oats' alone! Values for men and women are not equal when it comes to sexuality.

This difference in values also applies to teenagers. A study has revealed that a significant number of teenage girls feel they are not free to decide when to have sex, or use contraceptives, and many end up pregnant as a result.

When I started dating boys I was ill-equipped to handle the circumstances. The thought of making my debut filled me with fear because it meant asking a boy to accompany me and I worried about kissing him. I was nervous. I didn't want to kiss boys but felt I had no choice. My Patriarchal Voice made me feel obliged to kiss a boy, if that was his desire, and kept me restrained, restricted and silent with men and boys.

Drawing on two surveys of teenage sexual behaviour, demographer Ann Evans of the Australian National University, said pressure from boyfriends, lack of confidence and sexual ignorance led to many girls having sex when they did not want to, and/or without adequate contraception.

A survey of 1324 teenagers who had fallen pregnant found that two-thirds said they were unprepared for their first encounter and 18 per cent felt they were pressured or forced into having sex. Forty-five per cent of pregnant teenagers said that at some stage they had sex when they did not want to, mostly to please their partner or because they "had no choice".

When I was six years old I visited a neighbour's house to play. A man I didn't know appeared in the back yard. The kids said he was their uncle. I remember hearing them say he wasn't really an uncle, they just called him uncle. He came to me, put his arm around me and his hand up my dress. I stood helplessly restrained by his arm. He moved his finger in my vagina. I felt invaded and took the first opportunity to move away. I told no-one. Now I believe my Patriarchal Voice kept me silent. Perhaps the feeling was no-one would believe me and my Patriarchal Voice persuaded me I wasn't really hurt. How many women can relate to this? How often are women's experiences discounted by statements that women lie and make up stories about their treatment by men? I'm sure you would have heard the edict that women lie.

Differences in values extends to the names allotted to men and women who engage in sexual activity. There is an expectation that men are supposed to be highly sexed and it is normal for men and boys to act upon their urges. Women are not so privileged. Women who have sex outside the boundary of marriage are often belittled. A woman labelled a whore is so named not only by men's Patriarchal Voices but also by that same voice in women. Other derogatory names for women include Slut, Tart, Bit of Fluff, Floozy, Trollop, Bitch, Bird, Chick, Gold-digger, Bimbo, Biddy, Moo, Sheila and Luv.

Parts of women's bodies are also named disparagingly, for example Snatch, Cunt, Pussy, Boob, Knockers, Tit, Twat. A man's penis has many names, most are terms of endearment. Words that speak unkindly of a man's penis don't come easily to mind, except perhaps Prick. Can you think of any others?

4

Maintaining the System

"Anytime we see God as the male, rather than seeing God in all of us, we are cementing traditional thinking."

Anita Roddick <u>Business As Unusual</u>

The Patriarchal Voice passes from generation to generation through men and women. It is actually the women who reinforce its decrees. The system of control set up by the patriarchy is extremely successful. The Patriarchal Voice (inner) repeats and echoes patriarchal ideas (outer). Patriarchal authorities in religion, family, society, government and the media reinforce ideas of male supremacy. Feminine women are devalued and used rather than respected as equal human beings with equally valuable feminine qualities. Women are controlled by the patriarchy and they perpetuate the system by succumbing to the persuasions of the Patriarchal Voice in their heads. They allow the Patriarchal Voice to influence their thinking to excess and then they pass on these teachings to their children.

My grandfather died when my mother was two years old leaving my Grandmother, Anastasia, to raise five children. She lived on in their three bedroom house with her father-in-law. The patriarch occupied the front room, she shared a double bed in the second room with the two girls and the three boys slept in the third bedroom.

Anastasia owned several acres of land in Cheltenham and my mother's two brothers worked the land. They found huge deposits of sand. Twenty years after Anastasia bought the land the boys bought it from her for the very same price she paid. They mined the land for its sand and made their fortune.

My mother's sister stayed at home and looked after Anastasia till she died at age seventy-three. The house was sold and the money divided equally among the five offspring. My aunt who cared for her mother till her death received the same money as my uncles who now owned the farm. My aunt found herself without a home so she moved in with us. In the Patriarchal society most women were expected to work in the home and serve the family.

Inheritance is often left to males with little or nothing left to females. The Patriarchal Voice upholds and reinforces the ideas that men need money and property to care for the women in their lives, so women don't receive experience of handling money and property and often, as a result, appear ineffectual in dealing with finances.

I was the first of six children, three boys and three girls. When I was born my parents adored me. For sixteen months the sun shone on me, then my brother was born and everything changed. It was subtle at first and then I began to notice. I felt less important than my brother. He was 'son and heir' and being male was fed first, served larger helpings on bigger plates. The men were important and had priority. The boys believed that cleaning was women's work and it was a woman's job to serve. She was responsible for nourishment of body and soul (family relationships). Men were expected to work outside home, provide for family and take care of women.

Patriarchy and Religion

My father looked after us well. He was a good and gentle man who did his best as he knew. He absorbed the teachings of the patriarchal church. He listened to his friend, an Irish catholic priest, with whom he spent many happy hours playing tennis, and heeded his advice. My mother (covertly) and the priest (overtly) strongly carried patriarchal energy and my father, a university graduate, was not as staunch. My father probably suppressed his Patriarchal Voice because of the ardent patriarchal energy expressed by the people close to him. Two brothers fervently expressed the Patriarchal Voice and spoke disparagingly of women, "Their place is in the kitchen serving men. If women go beyond their god-given roles they are sluts and whores. Their opinions are idle." I quickly learned not to engage in discussions with those brothers whose ideas were so different from mine. The Church, a strongly patriarchal system, taught its members to uphold the status quo. The rules made insisted upon it with the pain of hell promised to anyone who dissented.

Martin is a disciple of religion. Speaking with his Patriarchal Voice he told me: *"The Patriarch refers to God. God writes on to my conscience the command to know Him, love Him and serve Him as His church teaches. Intuition tells me if I accede to that I will have done what I'm required to do to fulfil the purpose of my life, namely to achieve the beatific vision that is the presence of God after the moment of my inevitable departure from space and time."* Martin follows what the Church teaches believing that the rules and attitudes are God's direction and therefore 'infallible'. He believes if he chooses a different path he would suffer in the after-life.

The Church is a major influence on the thinking of its followers. My father absorbed what he heard from the pulpit and knelt to pray each night before bed. The patriarchal church had many Irish priests who influenced us with their philosophy. Dad's friend, the priest, advised him on many matters. He persuaded my father on where he should live (within walking distance of the church), how he should relate to my mother (not allow her too much authority) and how he should raise his children (children must obey their parents). According to the Church men are important and are suitable to be ministers of the Church. Women have less value and may not be ordained, but they may do jobs like playing the organ, assisting with fund raising, cleaning the sacristy or arranging the flowers. When I visited Ireland some years ago I clearly saw my Irish heritage in the Catholic culture. I observed pregnant women who already had large families, young girls with babies in their arms begging on the streets, and priests whose presbyteries were tended and cared for by women. These women bowed their heads and said, "Yes, Father", "No, Father." I also met an old grandmother who complained to the priest she felt useless because she could no longer work.

While writing this book I had a dream and this is what I recorded: *I'm in a church group of women and I don't know what I'm doing there. We are supposed to be outside and we are inside. I spend time with two of the members. My mother is one of them. They are totally strange (estrange) to me. I feel frustrated, helpless and lost. At one stage I see my mother running the big group. She seems to be doing very well. I hadn't realised she was so good at it. She is cool, calm, authoritative and clear. Some of the women dithered and didn't make it to the group. We were divided by not being able to get together.*

In this dream I clearly felt the energy of the patriarchy in my mother who was leading the group. The patriarchy comes through her (in an estranged way) and she is very good at teaching me the inner (covert) way. This dream confirmed for me that patriarchal energy, as taught by the church, is internalised and carried by women. We are divided in ourselves.

Like many of us you may have heard the following instructions given me by the Patriarchal Voice in my mother and the patriarchal church (nuns and priests) as I grew up.

"The man is the head of the house."
"Children should be seen and not heard."
"Honour your father and your mother."
"The man's name comes first. Write Mr & Mrs."
"The woman takes the man's name when she gets married and gives up her own. (The marriage probably won't last if she keeps her own name.)"
"Women are the weaker sex."
"Women and children need protection."
"Men's role is to protect women and children."
"Women serve men."
"Dress modestly."

When I started playing tennis with boys from a nearby college my mother cautioned me, "You must always let a man win." Years later when I was playing singles against a man and beating him my Patriarchal Voice reminded me to let him win. I watched myself hit balls into the net and out of the court. I felt powerless. My male opponent won the match.

A young woman told me her mother advised her regarding relationships with men, "You must pretend to be weak."

The Patriarchal Voice in Literature

A well-known children's story demonstrates how we unconsciously indoctrinate our offspring. The story of Jemima Puddle Duck by a female author subtly educates for patriarchal control. Beatrix Potter has written a story about a duck she calls a puddle duck – this implies that she puddles in life or swims in puddles that are not clean, clear or large bodies of water. Jemima allows herself to be seduced by a fox. She appears foolish and gullible and naive. Jemima does not have permission to sit on her own eggs (who said?) and when she subsequently is allowed to hatch out some eggs she is labelled a 'bad sitter' because her production rate is not 100%. Women and their work are trivialised in this story.

I read the popular Harry Potter books, the first of the series written in 1997, by J. K. Rowling (a woman). There is a pervasive sense of male supremacy and maintaining the 'status quo'. Women are portrayed sometimes as gossips and often at the mercy of their feelings. One wizard is called Hagrid (a hag is defined as an ugly old woman). I invite you to read other children's stories and gauge for yourself the subtle way we are unconsciously forming and perpetuating our young people's thinking.

Consider also the opinions so beautifully portrayed in My Fair Lady. Although perhaps exaggerated, Professor Higgins, Colonel Pickering and Alfred Doolittle's attitudes are not far from the actual truth in practice.

Patriarchal Indoctrination

Recently my mother had her hip replaced and needed extra care. My sisters are nurses and each moved in at different times to look after her. Sitting with my mother one day she looked at me and her Patriarchal Voice said: "You're very lucky!" I soon understood what she meant. If my sisters had not taken care of her, it would have been my responsibility. Part of me screamed inside me, "What about my brothers?" Perhaps you've noticed a similar situation where an elderly parent needs care. It usually falls to the daughters to predominantly look after them. There is not the same expectation of sons.

My mother was invited to lunch at my brother's. She commented to my sister it was a long way for my brother to drive her home, the implication being my sister could collect her instead. The distance was the same for both. My mother (with her Patriarchal Voice in charge) minimised the drive's importance for my sister and maximised it for my brother.

I'm tuned into patriarchal energy now. Becoming aware has been hard work. Because the Patriarchal Voice operates in shadow it's not overt. We may miss the subtlety. In this world where 'equality' is an important concept the ideas of the patriarchy are maintained and reinforced invisibly and covertly. That is why it is so hard to recognise. Our aim is to raise consciousness so we really do have choice.

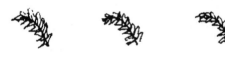

5

The Patriarchal Voice in Society

"Encouraged by business interests and the driving force of the pragmatic American consciousness, we insult the feminine at every turn."

Robert Bly <u>The Maiden King</u>

The patriarchy is the world being run according to men. Ideas passed down through generations in favour of men. For example, most primary positions in society are held by men. Men are honoured, listened to and obeyed. Women are a poor second.

With the rise of feminism men have become afraid women will take over and many men fear losing their power. They want to maintain control of women.

Beneath this fear do men believe women are more powerful? Possibly. Years ago, in a lecture, I was informed that women have a greater capability to survive alone than men - they are connected to an internal support system and most can more easily go within and get spiritual nourishment. I now think it could be because women are allowed to express their emotions, whereas men are not socialised in the same way and are more likely to need nurturing from someone outside themselves. Generally women really don't need men in order to manage. With advances in technology women can even conceive without a man. Basically men need women. Generally women live longer than men.

In Business

The patriarchy has traditionally devalued the work and the contribution of women. Many men have taken what women give and often not appreciated their worth. It is the unnoticed Patriarchal Voice that advises women and men to maintain the status quo.

Some years ago, I answered an advertisement for a pharmacist. The proprietor said: "I don't know. I've never worked with a lady." I replied: "Well, I'm not a lady. I'm a woman as distinct from a man." He agreed to see me.

I watched a woman working in an office with a man. He was official, officious and bossy. She ran around waiting on him, serving him and being pleasant. Her Patriarchal Voice kept her amenable. My awareness of her unconscious submission to her Patriarchal Voice made me feel uncomfortable.

Women who strive to succeed in business in a man's world often have to become masculine in thought and action. Energy follows thought and form follows energy. These women embody patriarchal energy. You may have noticed women who climb the corporate ladder have sometimes done so by emulating men. They must surrender many of their feminine ways, for example, dressing in power suits. If they don't emasculate they risk losing their status and may remain in a lower position in the corporate hierarchy.

The Patriarchal Voice often tells women who succeed in the business and corporate arena they have little chance of finding and keeping a man. They may be successful in one area but they are doomed to dismal failure in another. It believes a woman is not a 'real' woman without a man.

In Sport

Sponsorship is readily available for men's sport but not for women's sport. Even though the Australian Women's Hockey team won three gold medals at the 2000 Olympics Telstra withdrew sponsorship.

At the recent Olympics held in Sydney I noticed the females were given kisses from those presenting medals. The males received hand-shakes. Why is a woman expected to kiss strangers when a man need only shake hands? I heard the Patriarchal Voices of people in the audience objecting to flowers being given to all medal winners. The implication was it wasn't 'right' for men to receive flowers. Receiving flowers is a 'woman thing' and not something a 'real' man should do.

Social Effects

The Patriarchal Voice in women speaks from the shadows. It operates outside their awareness. The voice directs and they respond. They often don't realise they are acting in a way that may be counter to what they really believe. Many women find the battle with this inner unconscious voice so difficult they resort to taking antidepressant tablets. They know they feel depressed but because the voice is unconscious they may not know what to do to overcome it. Many more women than men are on antidepressants.

Thanks to the Patriarchal Voice many women find it difficult to acknowledge their value. I listened recently as a woman asked a mother of seven, "What do you do?" The mother replied, "Nothing." Relationships are not seen as important compared with paid employment.

A patriarch can be fair, just, wise and a firm decisive leader. I'm sure you know a patriarch who is a loving, generous father who epitomises these qualities. We can all benefit from using patriarchal energy appropriately and in balance in our personality.

It is when we deny its existence and don't honour its power and authority that the energy becomes destructive and acts out in ways which hurt self or others. For example, a woman climbing the corporate ladder may have to disown her feminine side and take on patriarchal energy. She may move ahead in the company, but at a price. She may display masculine traits and lose touch with her softer, vulnerable side that can connect with the inner essence of another. As a result her personal relationships could suffer.

A woman who listens to her Patriarchal Voice and still keeps her feminine power while climbing the corporate ladder can be personal and also be impersonal as well. She can be gentle and warm and also be firm when necessary. She can be receptive and directive as needed. She can be and do.

A man who honours his feminine side, while also honouring the Patriarchal Voice, can be a fair, firm, loving leader. He can protect. He can listen and share feelings. He can set boundaries and limits. He can make decisions and act on them. He can do and be.

6

He Who Must Be Obeyed

"A problem can never be resolved at the level of the problem, nor a paradox at the level of the paradox. One must rise above the level of the problem or the paradox to find a solution."

W. Brugh Joy M.D. Joy's Way

The Patriarchal Voice is the embodied voice of the patriarchy passed from generation to generation for six thousand years. This sub-personality carries the traditions and values of the ancient patriarchy. The Patriarchal Voice, operating in the mind, expresses the ideas and rules of the dominant philosophy of the patriarchal system. Usually we think it is who we are. We don't realise we have adopted this voice, or sub-personality.

The patriarchy is dominant in society and that's the position the Patriarchal Voice holds. Generally women are seen as inferior.

Because the patriarchy elevates men above women, so does the Patriarchal Voice. In fact it belittles women and trivialises who they are, what they stand for and what they do.

Most men are physically stronger than women. Throughout history men used their superior strength to dominate women. If women did not comply they often suffered at the hands of men. Even today in societies like the Taliban and in Afghanistan women suffer appalling atrocities and may even be shot if they disobey rules.

The patriarchy can also operate protectively as well as destructively. In the inner world the Patriarchal Voice develops as a form of protection. The Patriarchal Voice in women knows that women suffer if they don't obey patriarchal edicts and so it protects women by making sure they stay in the bounds of safety as defined by the patriarchal system. If they go against the dominant philosophy they may not be safe. It's often easier to obey the Patriarchal Voice, even though it may be to their disadvantage. For example, a woman obeys her Patriarchal Voice because it knows how to keep her safe, even though its protestations may hold her back or belittle her. Because this voice is unrecognised she hears it and complies. It influences her thoughts, feelings and deeds. The voice developed as a protection. Even though women have made great strides towards equality they are still being restrained by an invisible force. It's a paradox - the voice that restricts her also protects her.

Even today this unseen energy protects women. As much as they would choose not to be held back it is indoctrinated in them and on occasions necessary. Generally men are dominant and it is usually not wise for a woman to act as if she is as powerful as a man. Power is defined as 'the ability to do'. Women are often their own worst enemies as they fight a battle within themselves. The Patriarchal Voice tells them they cannot achieve without a man's help. If they accept this they lose their power. If they fight it they are still reacting to an internal energy that is in charge of their lives and they are not free to relate naturally to men.

It's in the heads of men and women but it supports men so it doesn't pose the same problem for men as for women. The rules are the same as those set up in the outer patriarchy. In the external world men have a different agenda from women. Similarly, in the inner world the Patriarchal Voice speaks to us differently from the Matriarchal Voice. The inner patriarch has a different set of rules from the inner matriarch. He cares about achievement, law and order. She looks to feelings and nurture.

I'm sure that, like me, you have met many a person who has a strong Patriarchal Voice. When the Patriarchal Voice is dominant it's as if patriarchal energy is in charge in the personality. The over-riding voice that speaks echoes the attitudes of the patriarchy.

You may be able to recognise this voice in people you know and as you read about people who have zealous inner patriarchs.

The inner patriarch has an ambivalent attitude towards women. Phillip who has a strong Patriarchal Voice usually doesn't like women. Of course, there is a part of Phillip that does like women, however his pro-women

67

voice is very weak. Phillip's Patriarchal Voice denigrates women's sexuality. It says women are absurd because they flirt with men and can seduce them. It speaks even more disparagingly of women who give their bodies freely to men maintaining this is unwise behaviour. Phillip's Patriarchal Voice doesn't have strong opinions when it comes to men giving their bodies away freely to women. It judges women, not men.

Dennis' Patriarchal Voice also expresses opinions about women. Here are some of its comments: *"Women's job is to look after men. They should stay in the home and take care of it. They should serve men - men do not do servile tasks in the home. Women serve men.*

Raising children is a woman's job. Men provide money and women do whatever is needed in the house to look after the men and the children. Men are important. They are the decision makers. Their ideas are valuable. Women's ideas are insignificant. Women are there for men. Men need to be looked after so men protect and care for women so women can do their duty."

Dennis' inner patriarch sees women as weak. He continues: *"Their brains don't function properly. What they say doesn't matter, it's basically flawed anyway and it doesn't always make logical sense. The Church is important. It's run by men and men rule. Women are only there to serve men. They're not equal. They must not be allowed to rise up or be given positions of power. Who knows what they would do? Who knows what foolish* ideas they would have? They wouldn't keep men in charge. They would want women to run the show. We cannot allow that. No way! Be wary of women. You must honour your mother and your wife, but you must not let them be superior. Don't give way to them. They are irrational, illogical, stupid creatures. Women's work is unpleasant! Cleaning and cooking is a necessary evil. Servile jobs should not be done by men. Labouring is okay but not servile house jobs. Labouring keeps a man's body fit and strong. That's valuable.

Women as sexual objects - urrrgh! They seduce men and make them weak. I don't like women. They must be denied. Women must be kept in their place. They must do as they are told. It is okay to use force if necessary. Women should hide their sexuality. They must not be showy or suggestive. Sex must be hidden."

Dennis' Patriarchal Voice has a lot to say and says it with passion. Similarly Mark's Patriarchal Voice maintains a woman's place is in the home. Mark's Patriarchal Voice says: "Women are made to bear children and raise them. Women are for man's pleasure and man's relief. They are only necessary because they bear the children. We must look after them for that reason. Women are made for giving men pleasure. Women must remember why they are here and do whatever is needed to care for the man, making sure he feels nurtured, satisfied, cared for, looked after, honoured, appreciated, acknowledged and obeyed."
The Patriarchal Voice trivialises women and their work.

In these men we hear reinforcement of the patriarchy. These voices are dominant and not operating from the shadows as often happens in women. I've used these examples here so we can see what a dominant Patriarchal Voice could say. These same ideas could be expressed in the head of a woman even though the voice does not appear to be dominant. Although not obvious in a woman it may still be dominant. Let us now tune in to a Patriarchal Voice of a woman.

Marcia's Patriarchal Voice has this to say: *"I exist in Marcia to take care of her, to protect her. She needs to be protected. She isn't able to do it for herself. She is weak, feeble, misled, easily taken advantage of, foolish, inappropriate, wild and a victim. I don't like her weakness. I don't like it when men take advantage of her. If she puts herself in a compromising situation and gets hurt I get upset. I'm determined to protect her."*

At the same time, Marcia's Matriarchal Voice says: *"I don't trust men. I see how they treat women. She allows men to take advantage of her, to use her, not to respect her or honour her. I tell her, he wants you for the sex. He'll use you and he doesn't really love you. He treats you well today, but what about tomorrow?*

If I see a man cry, I tell her he's weak, he cries too much. I see them look old and I tell her, he's too old. I feel so strongly about her relationship with men I make sure she doesn't get into any close relationships. I decide no man is good enough for her. That way she will always be single - and she will be safe!"

It's interesting that while Marcia's Patriarchal Voice prevents her from having a close relationship by pointing out her flaws, her Matriarchal Voice points out the imperfections in the men she meets. This plan ensures she never gets close enough to a man to have a committed relationship with him.

Let's look at some more statements. Perhaps you may have heard some of them before.

In a woman the Patriarchal Voice may say:
"A woman needs to be with a strong rational man."
"A woman is responsible for relationship. It's your fault he isn't feeling well."
"Don't go to sleep before he does."
"You must be available as soon as he arrives."
"Make sure he has finished speaking before you say anything."
"You mustn't be too sexual."
"You mustn't incite a man."
"Don't be too powerful."
"You must let him win."
"Don't trust a woman."
"Don't take up too much space."
"Don't become too prominent."
"You're too old to ... (dance, run, wear that, go alone, go out, sing.)"
"Stay in the background. Make yourself invisible."
"A woman doctor (dentist, broker, solicitor, hairdresser, chef ...) is not as good as a male doctor (dentist, broker, solicitor, hairdresser, chef ...)"

"It doesn't matter what you wear. There won't be any men there."

"You'll be a slave if you go into a relationship."

"You give up your freedom when you get married."

"You're not good enough to wear pearls."

"If you're given the money you'll probably meet a gigolo who will piss it away for you."

"Women are cursed - they bleed each month. They're unclean."

"Women bear children in pain. They have painful periods."

"Your vagina smells."

"A man doesn't want to know how you feel."

"You're only a ... housewife, mother, wife, woman, secretary, nurse."

"Woman driver!"

"She doesn't work. She's a mother."

"Mutton dressed up as lamb."

"You stupid bitch."

"Slut!"

"Floozy."

Sound familiar? The Patriarchal Voice echoes these thoughts inside your head just like a real person outside yourself. You may respond as if to a powerful person's pronouncements.

The implication behind these ideas is that women are not to be trusted, they are not capable, they are not as good as men, they are insignificant, they cannot look after themselves, they are not okay the way they are, their work is not important and their feminine qualities are not as valuable as masculine traits.

I was buying a house and considered choosing between recommended male and female brokers for finance. My Patriarchal Voice suggested a man is more experienced and effective than a woman. I chose the man and passed on the other recommendation (the woman) to a friend. The male broker gave me little information, my friend was given more facts and options from her female broker. As I asked for more information I found myself saying (in response to nagging from my Patriarchal Voice): "I know I'm being pushy". Because the broker wanted to veneer over detail, I felt intrusive. My loan cost 0.3% per annum more than my friend's. I wondered if my broker was receiving a large incentive from the bank.

We've looked at expressions of the Patriarchal Voice in women. Now let's examine how the same voice sounds in a man. In a man the Patriarchal Voice may say:
"Women's work is low value."
"You're not going to let a woman beat you, are you?"
"Don't let a woman take over."
"Don't show any feelings."
"Stay in control."
"No wonder she wanted you to pay."
"That's a woman's job."
"Men must be in charge of women."
"You're playing like a girl."
"Thank God you're not a woman."

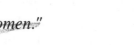

73

The implication behind these words is that a man must be strong, controlled and in charge. He must not show any weakness or vulnerability. If he shows a failing he risks being given the derogatory label of 'girl' or 'female'. How often have you heard a man labelled a 'woman' if he refrains from retaliating when his strength or honour is questioned? Commonly on the football field and other sporting arenas a man is expected to show aggression. If he appears weak he risks being called a 'girl' or 'an old woman'.

It is important to realise the words are not the only concern. The energy used makes the words important. It is the energy behind the words that gives them authority.

For example, at the airport a car driven by a woman was suddenly boxed in by a vehicle setting down passengers. As they were still unloading, the woman asked the driver if he would shift his car a little so she could exit. He made a move to grant her request. A woman with him said: "Stay there!" Her Patriarchal Voice spoke authoritatively knowing women can wait and women comply. I wonder would her voice have spoken thus if a man made the request?

A woman buying a packet of condoms and a card asked if she could borrow a pen. "It's for a joke," she explained. A man standing at the counter quipped: "Next thing you'll be trying to say you're a virgin." Her Patriarchal Voice made her justify her purchase to a stranger. His Patriarchal Voice permitted him to invalidate her.

74

After lunching with friends a woman departed saying: "I want to be home for my husband at a reasonable time. He lets me come out to lunch and I don't want to upset him." Her Patriarchal Voice reminds her she is a woman in a relationship to serve her man.

It requires time and effort to raise our awareness of our Patriarchal Voice. The concepts are ingrained and subtle. You and I need to be constantly alert to the voice and then we are better able to choose when to and when not to heed its pronouncements.

7

How the Patriarchal Voice
Influences Women

"The Inner Patriarch trivialises our gifts - at best, at worst - he shames us for possessing them."

Sidra Stone Ph.D. <u>The Shadow King</u>

Femininity is undervalued by the patriarchy. We are deprived of the right to enjoy and luxuriate in our feminine gifts. We are certainly not encouraged to enjoy being female.

The Patriarchal Voice speaks in women with a powerful energy to keep women from harm. The Patriarchal Voice says women must obey the rules of the patriarchal society to be safe. When a woman attempts to go beyond the boundaries set out for her by the ruling patriarchy, a man or a woman using patriarchal energy will put her in her place by opposing her, emotionally, physically or verbally. For their own survival, safety and protection women's Patriarchal Voices instruct women so they are pre-warned and protected. For example, many women find it hard to speak up for themselves in the work situation. If they do they risk losing employment. The results of an ACTU survey of 1000 women published in September 2001 stated women's main concern was job security. Most women already feel the judgements of their Patriarchal Voice holding them back so they are often in a weakened position before they attempt to speak out.

Women and Power

An area of concern for the Patriarchal Voice in women is the issue of power. A woman must not become too powerful. The Patriarchal Voice causes women to kill their power.

That we create life and nourish a baby in our wombs is not given full acknowledgment. This incredible power is not fully appreciated. Despite advances in science this still cannot be done effectively without a woman's body. Laboratories cannot come anywhere near growing a live healthy baby. God knows they've tried. What power that would be for the patriarchy! If this wondrous, natural, creative act by women is trivialised it is little wonder that what follows in nurturing and raising a child with the traditionally feminine gifts of caring and love is also undervalued.

Not only that, just as a woman has the power to begin a life she also has the power to end a life by stopping a pregnancy. Again, this is huge power that had to be negated by invalidating the right of a woman to choose whether to bear a child. Patriarchal society has fought long and hard to keep women under control by making abortion a legal and moral issue.

America's President Bush has a policy against abortion. This really is about control, keeping women in the United States subdued so their power is weakened.

The Patriarchal Voice subjugates women by denying them the knowledge they have this incredible power. Many don't even realise they have a life/death authority. Women can create and they can kill. They can end a life before anyone else knows about it. Of course, the Patriarchal Voice will probably make them feel guilty if they exercise this power. It could say, "Shame on you," or something stronger such as, "Murderer!"

It is okay for men to kill. Wars are justified. Abortions are not.

Many societies operate on the idea 'an eye for an eye'. The pay-back system justifies killing. It is not considered to be immoral for members of these cultures to retaliate by taking a life in return.

World leaders (patriarchs) can make a decision and drop a bomb or send an army to battle taking many lives. Winston Churchill (the patriarch) gave orders for Australian men to sacrifice themselves at Gallipoli.

As with all systems the person who holds the power is in a position to abuse it and it seems inevitable that a misuse of power occurs. The wise use of power becomes extraordinarily difficult and the thought of being without power causes fear in the one who holds dominion.

Throughout history people who have power have misused it. The pendulum swings and the weaker get stronger and rise up as we see happening with the changes caused by the women's movement. In the modern patriarchal society women are claiming their rights.

There is a saying, "Where power is women are not." Women must be willing to be powerful. Because we bear scars from the ways men have used their power over us, women often want no part of power.

Petra Kelly in
<u>Business As Unusual</u> Anita Roddick

In fact women have huge power. They can create and destroy life. The Patriarchal Voice within (and without) keeps this knowledge from women. Systems of control exist around giving birth and around aborting foetuses. To keep control it was necessary to make abortions illegal. The strongest and most persistent anti abortion voices come from the patriarchal churches.

Women have to accept being powerful and learn to use power. They need to be educated both within the home and the school to embrace power.

A large advertisement for a top class restaurant appeared in the daily newspaper. It read: "A gourmet who thinks of calories is like a tart who looks at her watch." I rang to speak to the woman responsible for placing the ad. and explained that I found it offensive. Later advertisements for that restaurant were different. When you notice a similar situation don't be afraid to speak out or take action. Events which seem insignificant can change the consciousness of those who are not aware.

Many women are confined and cannot allow themselves to say what they want. I was serving refreshments at a wake recently. I asked some older ladies: "Would you like a cup of tea?" Each replied: "Are you making one?" Their Patriarchal Voices gave them permission only if they were not being a bother, whereas men may say yes or no without having to qualify their decision.

Recently I talked to a woman who told me that in the early 1900's many women had their teeth removed as a gift to their future husband so they wouldn't create extra expense after the marriage.

Women and Other Women

Why are women suspicious of other women? Because mothers unconsciously pass on the legacy of the Patriarchal Voice. How many mothers have told their daughters not to trust another woman? Many a time I've heard it said: "Watch out for other women. If you tell her she'll pass it on to him. Don't trust her."

When a woman partner goes away on holiday or business the man is often invited to dinner. When a man goes away the woman usually does not receive a dinner invitation. Why is this? Why are women more inclined to ask a solo man than a woman to dinner? Do they think a woman can look after herself, whereas a man needs *cut down to size*

looking after? Does a woman fear competition from the other woman? Does the Patriarchal Voice say a woman is not worth bothering about? What do you think?

Sisters

Australian women are in even greater danger of undermining their 'sisters' because of our tendency to 'cut down tall poppies'. The Patriarchal Voice has had little opposition from the majority of Australian women in the past.

When promoting my book <u>The Intuitive Voice</u> I led a seminar at Border's book store. I told a friend and added: "Joan Kirner spoke last week." Joan Kirner succeeded in Australian politics and wrote a best selling book. My friend replied: "I don't have much time for her. She doesn't impress me." The Patriarchal Voice is powerful in many Australian women as this statement exemplifies. Whether my friend liked or approved of Joan Kirner was incidental to the fact that she was a successful and powerful woman. The point I'm making here is this. I was feeling good about presenting in a forum where other powerful people were speaking. With a quick statement my woman friend cut us both down to size. I'm sure this tendency is not restricted to women. Men are guilty of levelling other men. It is an Australian quality that is not diminished because it is also done by women.

Women and 'Sorry'

The Patriarchal Voice makes women apologise. Have you noticed how often women apologise? You may be surprised when you tune in to how regularly women use the word 'sorry'. It's not a word you hear often used by men. When I hit up at tennis in a team of women the most common word is 'sorry'. They apologise when they miss a shot, when they miss-hit the ball, when it crosses into the next court or hits the fence or the net.

Recently I was playing tennis with a woman who apologised when she could not get to a ball. If I lost a point she apologised for misleading me or for not encouraging me and she even apologised for not hitting it herself. She constantly said what she should have done instead of accepting what she did. Imagine how hard life is with this inner communication. I recognised in her myself, before I became aware of my inner voices apologising for me. With this voice nagging at me I felt uncomfortable and depressed. Once I separated the Patriarchal Voice from my other inner voices and took charge myself life was more peaceful and joyful.

I'm concerned at repetition of the word 'sorry' because the dark side of this behaviour is that the person may eventually apologise for *being*.

Recently I was listening to a radio football commentary. Frequently the broadcast crossed 'around the grounds' to up-date scores. At one match a woman gave the tally. Her voice was a pleasant change from a man's. I noticed she used the word 'sorry' three times in as many minutes. She gave wrong details, immediately apologised and gave the right tally. Football is a man's area. Not only was she a woman being judged by men and women but her toughest critique came from her Patriarchal Voice.

inner critic

Women are disadvantaged because they must answer to an internal, invisible and exacting master. He is constantly nagging, making them over prepare, over perform and apologise for any perceived shortfall.

Women and Liberation

political forum for one's passion

Anita Roddick is an entrepreneur who created the Body Shop as a successful franchise system that now has branches all over the world. I believe she is a fine example of what a woman can bring to the world of business. She calls for business to assume a moral leadership and uses the Body Shop as a political forum for her passions. The following quote was displayed throughout the world in her outlets. We could attribute to the Patriarchal Voice many of the conclusions that it echoes in the heads of women and men.

double standards

"Because women's work is never done <u>and</u> is underpaid or unpaid or boring or repetitive <u>and</u> we're the first to get the sack <u>and</u> what we look like is more important than what we do <u>and</u> if we get raped it's our fault <u>and</u> if we get bashed we must have provoked it <u>and</u> if we raise our voices we're nagging bitches <u>and</u> if we enjoy sex we're nymphos <u>and</u> if we don't we're frigid <u>and</u> if we love women it's because we can't get a 'real' man <u>and</u> if we ask our doctors too many questions we're neurotic or pushy <u>and</u> if we expect community care for our children we're aggressive <u>and</u> 'unfeminine' <u>and</u> if we don't we're typical weak females <u>and</u> if we want to get married we're out to trap a man <u>and</u> if we don't we're unnatural <u>and</u> because we still can't get a safe, adequate contraceptive but men

can walk on the moon <u>and</u> if we can't cope or don't want a pregnancy we're made to feel guilty about abortion <u>and</u> for lots and lots of other reasons we are part of The Women's Liberation Movement ..."

Anita Roddick <u>Business As Unusual</u>

With the movement for Women's Liberation I took on the idea 'women are okay' and suppressed my Patriarchal Voice because it said, 'women are not okay'. We need to educate the patriarchal system to value women as women and men as men. They need not compete or be enemies. They can, and should, compliment each other and appreciate each other's value. Women have qualities that are different from those of men. Femininity has its own beauty as does masculinity. One has value as does the other, like night and day, black and white, inside and outside. They are different and each has value. Like Yin and Yang one is integral to the other.

Each person, whether male or female, benefits from a balance of masculine and feminine energies as Marion Woodman explains in the following extract.

"Viewed in the context of the divine marriage in both men and women, the subordination of the feminine to the masculine, outwardly enacted as the subordination of women to men, is a horrendous lie. For at least three thousand years women have carried, whether consciously or unconsciously, their culturally determined role in relation to men, an inferior role that has left their masculinity wounded by patriarchal

training. As a result of the inferior role assigned to the feminine, men are culturally and personally crippled by a weak feminine every bit as disabling as the weak masculine in women. As complimentary energies, masculinity and femininity require each other for natural balance in relationships. A weak feminine in men produces a distorted, one-sided masculine - the militarist, the corporate robot; a weak masculine in women produces a distorted, one-sided feminine - the baby doll, who pretends to be everything any man imagines her to be, or a Gorgon, who reduces others to stone."

Marion Woodman The Maiden King

Synergy in Women

Synergy is created when the behaviour of the whole is greater than the behaviour of the sum of its parts. Synergy magnifies situations. When the Patriarchal Voice combines with a woman's inner critic the effect is stronger by far. The inner critic of a woman constantly reminds her of her shortcomings, her looks, her weight, her actions. A man's inner critic is much less concerned about his looks, his weight, his actions or even his speech. The inner critic gives men a hard time about other things, for example his performance at work, his income, or the type of car he drives. The synergistic effect probably doesn't occur to the same extent in men because the Patriarchal Voice does not devalue masculinity.

Women and Loathing

love energy

Some women mistakenly believe the men who abuse them really love them. They may remain in relationship because they are sure they are loved. It doesn't register that love has turned to dislike. Germaine Greer, author of The Whole Woman, in the chapter entitled Loathing says: *"A few men hate all women all of the time, some men hate some women all of the time, and all men hate some women some of the time."*

This is true. In each person's personality, depending on which parts, sub-personalities or selves are in charge, there exists the possibility for love or hatred in all percentages. It therefore stands to reason that a few women hate all men all of the time, some women hate some men all of the time and all women hate some men some of the time. When love goes away something else, another force or energy, take its place. The other side of love may indeed be hatred or loathing.

The Matriarchal Voice

Matriarchs see value in women. They believe women are superior to men. They propose a society led by women as better than the one we have. My mother, as a matriarch, was uncomfortable with her lack of power in a man's world and her Matriarchal Voice said things like the following:
"Women are mentally and emotionally stronger than men."

"If women were running the world it wouldn't be in the mess it's in."
"Women can tolerate pain better than men."
"Men need women to care for them."
"Women live longer. They survive without a partner better than men."
"Women should design kitchens."
"Most men are really just little boys."

I'm sure you are familiar with some of these statements.

The Matriarchal Voice in men plays a similar role to the Patriarchal Voice in women. It speaks disparagingly of men and shames them for many male tendencies, such as being competitive, being sexual without feeling and being aggressive. If it is a traditional masculine trait it is denigrated, for example a statement like, "Men think with their penises." The Matriarchal Voice can give men a hard time. It usually does not present the same problems for men as the Patriarchal Voice does for women because it is not in alignment with the dominant culture.

Women Need to Love and Respect Themselves

The Bible states: "Love your neighbour as yourself." Many think this means love your neighbour. It means love yourself first and love your neighbour. Everyday I see examples of women who have little idea of the disservice they do themselves by overlooking their own needs. Their inner dialogue may actually be hurting them. The inner critic is hard on both men and women. It

Voiu bashiup

criticises women constantly on how they look and what they say and do. This voice repeating the same failings over and over is like child bashing as their inner child suffers from the constant barrage of complaints. Emotionally they are abused internally and sometimes this can lead to having in the external world a partner who physically, mentally or emotionally harms them.

A report in The New Idea June 23, 2001 entitled 'Could Your Man Become Violent?' by Alex Tate tells the story of a woman whose 'ideal' husband began to abuse and restrain her. Research from the Australian Bureau of Statistics Women's Safety Survey reveals that of all women who have been married or have lived with a partner 23% have experienced domestic violence, with 42% of these women pregnant at the time.

Many women also abuse their partners, but statistics are not so readily available.

It is our responsibility to become aware of the fact that our inner dialogue is not serving us and may be hurting us. When we take responsibility for our inner world this can lead to changes in our external world. When we make internal changes for the better (learn to respect ourselves) people we judged or blamed are no longer so much of a problem. They leave, we leave, or we learn a new way to deal with them.

Women need to learn to love themselves. For so long they have given everything to others - parents, work, children, partners. It is a common thing for women to give to others before they give to themselves. They see their mothers do it and they learn from this role-model. Loving yourself sometimes means saying no to others. When love goes sour in a relationship many women continue to suffer indignities for too long. This may not be a good role-model for their children.

The Patriarchal Voice is an inner saboteur who dislikes women. By bringing this energy to awareness we make conscious what was unconscious and we move forward on a journey to change women's and men's inner dialogues. *Instead of reacting, we need to embrace the Patriarchal Voice.* It then has a chance to change, transform and support women's empowerment rather than sabotage it.

8
How the Patriarchal Voice Directs Men

"Men are a mess. Our marriages fail, our kids hate us, we die from stress and on the way we destroy the world."

Steve Biddulph Manhood

Historically fathers worked alongside wives and children. The entire village raised the child. Then the Industrial Revolution took men and many children out of the family and put them to work in a factory or mine. From that time on most fathers have not been around to participate in raising the children. The Industrial Revolution broke the chain that taught men how to be 'men'. Men left home to go out to work and women began to raise the children without the assistance of males. In the past unless the tribe raised 'good' men the tribe and village were endangered.

The women's movement has made inroads into changing the way men and women relate. Women have changed and so have men. Many men have been involved in the women's movement. They know the old way of domination of male over female is losing its place in today's world. They have opened themselves to become SNAGS – Sensitive New Age Guys (even this name is derogatory). They may be more open to experiencing feelings. This exposes them to criticism from the patriarchy. In SNAGS the Patriarchal Voice is often suppressed and disowned.

In societies that remain strongly patriarchal, for example many Italian and Greek communities, the patriarch knows his place as head of the family and takes pride in honouring the role he inherited. Men with a strong Patriarchal Voice have a natural expectation of authority and privilege. They know their role, what to do and how to do it. Families without that strong heritage may lack clear direction. The men may be unsure of their authority and often suppress their inner Patriarchal Voice. Today many men feel lost. They wonder what role to take on to best guide their families. When men suppress the Patriarchal Voice they may be indecisive and lacking in a clear sense of direction. Many men are no longer sure who they are.

Feminism is supposed to be good for men. It upholds equality of opportunity and value of men and women. In fact, many men and women have felt oppressed by feminism. Perhaps a reason may be that there has not been a balance. Feminists have often gone too far in one direction without embracing the value of the opposite. Women's liberation is also men's liberation. As Steve Biddulph says in <u>Manhood</u>, "You can't liberate only half the human race."

While the Patriarchal Voice respects and promotes the power of men, their feelings are not something it knows a great deal about. Men suffer much grief and pain in their isolation. Men are often lonely and unhappy. The Patriarchal Voice is not comfortable expressing vulnerability so many men pretend they are okay and hide feelings of inadequacy.

Steve Biddulph says that by the nineties men displayed phoney toughness and phoney niceness. The Patriarchal Voice has standards. If men don't really demonstrate the toughness of their forebears this could appear as a weakness. With each thought and action the Patriarchal Voice then persuades men they are ineffectual and inefficient. This increases their feelings of failure and engenders a phoney niceness. Men often feel inadequate and lacking in direction and purpose and yet they have to be 'nice'. The Patriarchal Voice can rule wisely whether perceived as nice or not. It is not concerned with images of perception. The inner patriarch does what he does because he believes his role demands it.

It is becoming obvious that many men are feeling out of place as described in the following articles. As men open themselves to experiencing more of their femininity the perception seems to be they are becoming effeminate and that is inferior and 'not okay'.

This extract, written by a man, was unsigned and appeared in The Sun Sunday Magazine June 2000.
Are men the new women? Received wisdom insists that the male of the species is as unsuited for survival in the modern world as Tyrannosaurus (rex) at a Tupperware

93

party. We are seen as pathetic creatures, redundant sperm banks wandering the post-industrial wastelands like obsolescent missing links, our heads hung in shame at what we used to be. We're forced to eat in pastel-coloured cafes. We drive small feminine cars. Hell, even computers are looking girlie. Welcome to the new feminocracy where advertisers and TV sitcoms cast men as slightly ridiculous creatures unsuited to life in the modern world. Women are no longer the weaker sex, says Dylan Jones - caveman has turned into quiche man.

Michelle Griffin in The Age October 22, 2000 wrote: *"Once it was enough for a man to be, well, a man. These days, we're not so sure. Blokes are supposed to be sensitive, but should they wear moisturiser? Is it OK to drink beer with the boys? And is it possible to be a brilliant dad and still go places at work?"* While researching a story on child care she rang ten firms to find men who were working part-time to be with their children. She found none. The reason given was "career suicide". (Women at this level also experience career suicide and that's normal for women.) Men who take time out for children are more often self-employed. She concludes the men's movement "has only one extremely valid goal - to get blokes to talk to each other about what's going on in their lives."

In the article the assumption is made that men who join a men's group are usually at a crisis point. They attend because they realise they are not always in control. They learn to talk about their feelings and listen to others.

When they leave the safety of the group they usually don't talk about their experiences with their mates. I expect their Patriarchal Voices tell them feelings are women's business. If it is to do with women it is trivialised. They must be seen as manly.

Many men are suffering. They've lost their identity and sense of direction. Men I've met recently have admitted they are struggling. They ask who is a good role model for a man to follow? The men's movement has been delayed. It is now time for men to find out who they are in this new era.

Today many men have lost their ability to use their Patriarchal Voice with wisdom. Often single men wait for women to approach them, many have stopped the pursuit and given up the chase.

As the population of the world has increased there is no longer pressure to produce children to 'keep the tribe going'. Many men have abandoned the idea of partnering a woman and have chosen instead to publicly partner a man. We could ask, why not? Perhaps men understand other men and perhaps women better understand other women. A woman may know what another woman would desire for sexual fulfilment. Many people are accepting being labelled 'gay'.

Because a choice is made to partner someone of the same sex there is no escape from patriarchal energy. In a partnership when one disowns the Patriarchal Voice it is possible the other partner will express it and it may manifest in destructive ways, for example in addictions, authoritarianism or domination of one partner by the other. A couple who disowns patriarchal energy may draw in friends, extended family or work associates who express the energy as disapproval.

Most men take up more space than most women. Usually for men taking space is not an issue. Because of the influence of the Patriarchal Voice many women tend to contain themselves and often feel uncomfortable about space they occupy, whether it be physically or energetically. When men become gay and honour more of their feminine traits they also may apologise for taking up space. When women become gay they may not be so concerned with taking room for themselves. They may be noisier and bolder.

Women and men are different. Their energies have different vibrations. It is energy that vibrates in masculine ways and in feminine ways depending on the form. A man can vibrate with feminine energy and a female can vibrate with masculine energy. It is all energy. It has been a rule of the patriarchy to diminish the value of feminine energy so if a man chooses to demonstrate femininity in any form he may be assessed by his Patriarchal Voice as low-grade or pathetic.

The women's movement and the men's movement are having an effect, albeit perhaps superficially. The Patriarchal Voice in men and women is deeply entrenched and is resisting change. We need to become aware of this internal dialogue and then we have a chance to respond positively to the shifts.

―

9

So This Is Wot Wimmin Want?

Strewth!

By David Campbell
with kind permission.

In the style of C.J. Dennis' The Sentimental Bloke as he
might have tackled ... feminism. 'The bloke' can't
understand what's troubling Doreen, so he has a chat with
Ginger Mick ... with disturbing results.

> Yer know Doreen, fer oo me 'eart
> Was 'it by Cupid's flyin' dart,
> Well ... I dunno ... but lately she
> 'As seemed a bit ... well ... odd ter me.
> At supper, where she useter tork,
> She sits an' fiddles wiv 'er fork.
> She sighs a lot, an gazes out
> The winder. Wot's she on about?
> I tries ter keep orl cheerful-like
> An' 'elp 'er wiv the little tyke,
> But still she gets that starin' look,
> Which leaves me feelin' ... sorter crook!
> I 'as a word wiv Ginger Mick
> Cos 'e's me mate, an' knows a trick

Or two 'bout wimmin ... wot they think ...
An' 'ow ter keep em in the pink.
It seems ter me, 'e sez, Doreen
Is pinin' fer wot mighter been.
Geewhizz, I sez, I never did ...
Yer think she wants another kid?

Then Mick jus' sits an thinks a bit.
No mate, 'e sez, that sure ain't it.
These wimmin, see, they gets a yen
Ter 'ave a life ... well ... more like men.
Goorstrooth! That 'it me fer a six,
An lef' me in a proper fix!
Wot did it mean? I arst yer now ...
Me sweet Doreen be'ind a plough?
That carn't be it, I mean ter say ...
Wot skirt'd want ter spend 'er day
Wiv brakin' back an' achin' feet
Out in the rain an' scorchin' 'eat?
Don't get me wrong ... I dips me lid
Ter wimmin wot 'ave 'ad a kid.
That birthin' lark sure ain't no joke ...
I thanks the Lord that I'm a bloke!

But ... 'ere now ... lemme get this strate:
Instead uv waiting at the gate
Ter greet 'er man when day is done,
Shed rather swet out in the sun?

"Yer wimmin want," sed my ole Gran,
"An 'ouse, a kid, a decent man
'Oo'll come 'ome sober ev'ry night,
An' show respec' an' treat 'em right."
But wimmin now ...well, I dunno
Wot makes em tick, wot makes em go ...
An keep me guessin' wot comes nex' ...
It sure won't be wot I expecks!

I ain't much good wiv words an such,
An never likes to tork too much,
But Gawd! I'll 'ave to face Doreen
Ter see which bit uv grass is green.

We'll work it thro, I know we will ...
Jus' me, Doreen, an' little Bill.
It's somethin' I jus' gotta do ...
I couldn't live wivout them two!

I'll grab the bull fair by the 'orns
An' see wot's causin' orl them yorns,
Wot's 'id be'ind orl 'er sorrer,
An' I'll do it ... come termorrer!

Doreen's Patriarchal Voice prevents her from telling Bill
what is bothering her. Bill's Patriarchal Voice knows his
role, women's place and women's work, but is lost when
it comes to talking to Doreen about her feelings.

10

The Role of the Father

"The passive man may skip over parenting. Parenting means feeling, but it also means doing all sorts of boring tasks - taking children to school, buying them jackets, attending band concerts, dealing with curfew, setting rules of behaviour, deciding on responses when these rules are broken, checking on who a child's friends are, listening to the child's talk in an active way, etc. The passive man leaves his wife to do that."

Robert Bly in <u>Wingspan</u>

A girl child is often adored by her father. There may be a special connection between them. A mother cannot share this relationship. As the child reaches puberty she becomes sexually attractive and this attraction is off-limits. The father most often squashes the sexual urges he feels. He is probably not able to talk about this with his wife so he does his best to push the feelings away. He withdraws his energy from his special love. His daughter may not understand why suddenly she feels alone and abandoned by her father. Her first love affair (with her father) fails and she doesn't understand what happened.

Like me you may remember experiences with your father. I had a loving connection with my dad. I knew he cared deeply for me. I recall one day when as a young teenager I ran in and jumped on his lap as he sat in a chair. He pushed me away and I felt the pain in my heart. I didn't understand it. I felt hurt. After that our special connection seemed to be lost.

The positive side of a parent's Patriarchal Voice stands against invasion to protect both boys and girls. It guards them against being molested. But we give mixed messages. We tell our children: "Go and sit on Santa's knee." The negative side of a parent's Patriarchal Voice could allow invasion to happen. Many parents from patriarchal families believe they own their children's bodies. They may say: "They're my children." The emphasis is on ownership.

Fathers raising young girls often have a difficult time with their daughter's sexuality. Men must be able to raise daughters and still have clear boundaries between them. It's often even not appropriate for a father to talk 'sexy' or tell his daughter 'dirty jokes'. The gift of an appropriate Patriarchal Voice of a father by marriage (father-in-law) is that his new daughters can be protected with clear boundaries as he maintains distance between them.

Young girls may be very attractive to their fathers. The daughter is often in a quandary whether or not to resist her father if he is sexually inappropriate. If he sexually molests her she may be afraid to say no. She carries the blame. As a female, no matter how young she was, her Patriarchal Voice says if she hadn't lured him he wouldn't have done it.

When a young girl is attractive a father must maintain clear boundaries between them. If he violates this trust the Patriarchal Voice in the woman upholds the incest taboo and blames the woman. This could result in her becoming sexually frigid. She may not understand why she is restricted sexually. She is afraid to be seductive because her Patriarchal Voice suggests the incest was a result of her seductivity and therefore her fault.

A father can use a warm loving energy, with an open heart, and not violate the space between his daughter and himself. He can hold the space. He does not need to withdraw his energy.

Children often feel restricted by their parents. Young people don't have the freedom money brings. They are necessarily restrained. They may take on the dictates issued by the parental patriarchs (inner and outer) and internalise the rules.

When I was growing up there was little money to spare after feeding two parents, an aunt and six children so dad usually said no when I asked for extras or luxuries. That Patriarchal Voice is still in my head making me feel guilty when I spend money on indulgences for myself.

In most families the man is head of the house. However, the Patriarchal Voice is not always strongest in the male. My father was a humble man. He was not what is commonly known as a male chauvinist. He worked hard at the office, often going at lunch time to the market for fruit and vegetables that he would bring home for us. He made porridge for the family for breakfast frequently giving my mother and me breakfast in bed. While Mum cooked dinner Dad would wash and dry the dishes. When Mum developed problems with her knee Dad took over the clothes washing as well. He also vacuumed. He did what he believed needed to be done.

It was my mother who strongly articulated the Patriarchal Voice and Dad suppressed his. He took advice from his friend, the Irish Catholic Priest, who expressed his Patriarchal Voice as well. With this pair of strong Patriarchal Voices near him Dad didn't need to assert his.

When the women's movement was gaining momentum it became difficult for my dad, as a thinking man who had been to university and understood how women had been discriminated against, to uphold the position held by the patriarchy.

11
Helping Women To Become Helpless?

"The Inner Patriarch acts like the magician in the fairy tales, transforming a grown woman into a daughter. This daughter, in turn, transforms every man that she meets into a father and so subverts her own power."

Sidra Stone Ph.D. The Shadow King

Patriarchs can be good loving fathers. A caring father means well, but power is easy to misuse. The patriarchal society has kept women in the home 'for their own good'.

Without question women are usually not as physically strong as men. Men, of necessity, do many manual labour tasks that women cannot do. Historically men were the hunters and warriors. Women stayed at home and prepared the food. Women's chores were around the home including looking after children while men went out and brought home their prey.

Men fought enemies, often having to kill to protect their loved ones. The patriarchal society protects its women. Care and protection are given with loving intentions. The boundaries have been defined for centuries and it is within these limits that women are to stay, 'for their own good'.

It is difficult for women to step outside these boundaries. They've existed for six thousand years and women have been kept relatively safely within them.

The patriarchy believes women are inferior to men because they are physically weaker and it is accepted they are less able to achieve in the world of men. However, in recent years many great advancements in business have been made by women. They are reaching top positions, albeit these are in the minority, it *is* happening. A study released in January 2001 reveals that of the 7341 board positions in Australia, 251 are held by 155 women. Women occupy only 3.4 per cent of board positions in publicly listed companies. When asked why numbers of women board members were so low many of these women said men tended to promote each other. It's not easy for women to achieve high positions in traditionally a man's world. They do indeed have a challenging journey. Full equality is still a dream.

The Patriarchal Society makes a fuss about protecting women and looking after them. The assumption is they aren't capable themselves. If self-protection were fostered women could learn to take care of themselves. As they are instructed in helplessness the end product is women who believe they are unable to protect themselves. Women are not naturally helpless. They have been educated and controlled within the patriarchal system to believe this and their Patriarchal Voices have taken up the cause.

Recently I played tennis in a team against a dominant man. He talked constantly throughout the match. His wife was his tennis partner. His daughter waited impatiently to go home. Between rubbers I discovered how anxious she was. She was too scared to carry her cup (in case she spilled the contents) and to take herself to the lavatory. Our match was delayed while her mother accompanied her. I became aware how the father controlled those around him, his dominant attitude breeding fear and helplessness in his daughter and discomfort and rebelliousness in his wife.

Daughters are educated for helplessness by being told they need protection and by being socialised to be helpless. We are encouraged to get men to aid us. We're told it is important to make them feel needed and valued. Many a time I've accepted help instead of using my own resources. I'm not saying it isn't okay to accept help. I am saying our helplessness is fostered.

I'm often amazed when things happen in my environment that serve to teach me about issues I'm pondering. While out walking in the country one day I came across a group of young men kicking a football in the street. As I went past them I took one side of the road. I thought about men protecting women. Just then one of the guys kicked a football up in a tree and, in spite of the otherwise empty road, it landed down on me! I wondered what that was about. Was I being shown that women needed to take more responsibility to protect themselves?

I was still thinking about men protecting women a couple of days later and house-sitting alone while two front rooms were being renovated. The painters spent the day redecorating the rooms and planned to return the next day to paint the woodwork. At day's end the men left, without explanation, leaving the windows wide open to release the fumes, and the front door pulled to, with the lock open. Part of me (my inner child) felt scared. If I left my safety in their hands I was in a vulnerable situation. I closed the windows and locked the door.

Not only do situations arise to teach us, our dreams also offer insights. If we look at our dreams we may be able to see how the unconscious is communicating to reinforce understanding. I suggest you write down your dreams and re-read them to see what your unconscious may be telling you.

I had a dream:
I'm preparing to go to a ball and I realise I'll be cold coming home so I ask a friend to take a shawl to the restaurant for me. I wonder why I'm taking a baby's shawl to protect me when I'm wearing a black dress. The shawl is not at all suitable.

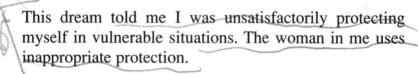

This dream told me I was unsatisfactorily protecting myself in vulnerable situations. The woman in me uses inappropriate protection.

In the growing up process we take on many energies, many ways of being. We choose the ones to best suit our purpose at the time. Women are led to believe that being

I Thought I Knew

feminine implies needing to be looked after. If men take on feminine energy, without the balance of a strong masculine (for example by becoming gay), they may also take on associated fears and helplessness.

Women get raped by men. Men are physically more powerful than women and some seem to feel that women are for their use. In The Whole Woman Germaine Greer says: "Women are raped, abused and harassed, not by rampaging strangers, but by men they see every day, men they thought they knew or men they thought they could ignore."

Women expect men to protect them. We've been encouraged to believe they will. *We must take responsibility for our own safety* and not leave it in the hands of others we think we can trust.

Currently, at the time of writing, there is discussion whether pregnant women should be banned from playing netball. Women are not allowed to make their own decisions. Power is exercised over women who are not encouraged or expected to understand their own bodies. At the same time on the news I see a woman eight months pregnant playing golf. The Patriarchal Voice might say, "Scandalous!" What did yours say when you read this?

In like manner that the patriarchy controls women in society it issues rules about making babies. We've been led to believe we are victims of our biology, that we are not in charge of our reproductive system. We've been led to believe conception is out of our hands and we need to take a birth control pill, or intervene in other ways, to prevent a sperm from fertilising an egg. What if we do have the power to choose whether to become pregnant or not? I believe we have more say than we realise. I believe women have this huge power and do not recognise it. As you read this you may think this is a strange idea. Years ago I read the book <u>Bringers of the Dawn</u> *Teachings of the Pleiadians* by Barbara Marciniak. It stated: *"They (those in control) convince you, by continuously putting these issues (abortion) before you, that a woman has no control over the birthing process in her body. You don't need abortion: you never need to get pregnant in the first place if you don't desire it. How? By will. A woman can say to herself, I am not prepared at this time for a child. Or, alternately, I am in receptivity of a child. When you own yourself, you will not need permission from the government about what you can do with your own body."*

As I considered this idea I came to see truth in it. I realised that I had conceived only the number of children I desired. I also noticed that some women who became pregnant, when it seemed inappropriate, actually wanted to conceive a baby for underlying psychological reasons. I'm sure you can think of examples of people who say they want children who don't conceive, and others who say they don't want children who become pregnant. It is not simple because there are so many factors to consider. Considering our conditioning in patriarchal society, I realise this is a radical idea. I'm merely raising it as a question. What if the patriarchy have been using the idea of controlling women's fertility to maintain their control over women? We may not know the whole story.

If parents use patriarchal energy in educating their children we could develop men and women who know how to take care of themselves and have the power to do so. The Patriarchal Voice, used with awareness, can say: "No." It can set limits and boundaries to protect. Women and men would be better equipped to safeguard themselves in times of risk.

When we raise patriarchal energy in ourselves it is unconsciously felt by others as a vibration. Others will not mess with us if we are in charge of our own energy domain. (See Chapter 19 Understanding Energy, Linkage and Flow.)

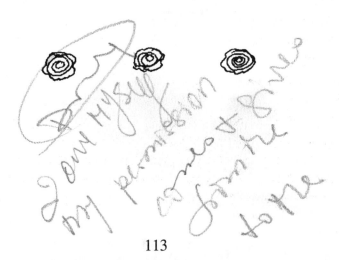

12

The Patriarchal Voice in the Health Industry

"A recent study of women's health and wellbeing set me thinking about the changes women have achieved in their lives over the past 40 or 50 years. All were absolutely necessary, but most of these changes seem to have been to women's external lives. The women's movement has had minimal impact on the inner world, it seems to me."

Dr Peter O'Connor Psychotherapist & Author

The Patriarchal Voice is at work in the health industry. It is a major force present in doctors, nurses and patients.

"In some future epoch intelligent beings from another galaxy will hold seminars to discuss possible explanations of why a whole generation of female earthlings had their bellies cut open.

Intellectual feminists have written millions of words on the ways in which men have colonised and controlled women but still the process rolls on, aided by better techniques for exploration and analysis and storage of data. Much of what is done to women in the name of health has no rationale beyond control.

115

Men have the right to take care of themselves, or not, as they see fit, but women are to be taken care of whether they like it or not. Screening is many times more likely to destroy a woman's peace of mind than it is to save her life. Women are driven through the health system like sheep through a dip. The disease they are being treated for is womanhood."

Germaine Greer <u>The Whole Woman</u>

The inner patriarch is responsible for women's lack of belief in their bodies. He makes them doubt their normal body function. At menstruation women buy tampons, many also buy tablets, naprogesic, ponstan and other anti-inflammatories, to ease discomfort of a natural body action.

Large numbers of women are having their wombs removed. These days the operation is performed through the vagina so there is no need to cut open the abdomen. I heard a woman say she had her womb removed because she found she couldn't take hormone replacement therapy. Why was she convinced she needed HRT? I believe the Patriarchal Voice in women is responsible for making them suffer during menstruation, childbirth and menopause. The voice totally convinces women there is something wrong with them.

A woman worried because her period seemed abnormal. She was nearing menopause and the bleeding was erratic and prolonged. (It's been my observation as a woman and a pharmacist that it's normal for periods to get heavier before menopause). Her male doctor wanted her to go on the pill (which did not suit her at nearly 52 years of age). He said: "Women used to die from that." ('That' was probably enough to make a vulnerable woman worried she was also in danger of death). The doctor's Patriarchal Voice attempted to control her. The female patient's Patriarchal Voice made her doubt her body's actions and reactions and pointed out that the blood did not look pleasant.

When women menstruate the lining of the womb leaves the body mixed with blood and fluids. This normal bodily function may cause discomfort and inconvenience. It is natural for a woman's body to retain extra fluid at certain times of the month. A few days later the kidneys usually excrete the excess fluid and her body returns to its previous state. At these times many women feel stress as their Patriarchal Voice reminds them of their 'weakness'.

Rachel Pollack states in <u>Seventy-Eight Degrees of Wisdom</u> *"Menstruation (the word 'menses' relates to 'month' and 'moon') is miraculous, because menstruating women bleed copiously yet do not die. Further, many women find themselves more emotional, but also more psychic when menstruating. Fearing this power, men have created disturbing myths and taboos around menstruation. But power does not have to be destructive or even frightening. If respected this lunar psychic awakening enriches life."*

Giving Birth

A picture in a women's magazine showing a woman late in her pregnancy bears the caption: "About to pop any day." The glorious, magnificent, incredibly creative process is trivialised by her own gender.

Women in labour apologise for making noise, for being a problem, for being needy and for not being in control. Their Patriarchal Voices make them feel guilty, uncomfortable and a nuisance. They remind women they are taking up time and space instead of efficiently and quietly producing a child.

Many men will not allow their wives pain control in child-birth. Some husbands (patriarchs) forbid epidural injections. The Patriarchal Voices in the wives undermine their own discomfort by causing them to comply.

Wives in birthing units with husbands who stay the night worry their husbands won't get enough sleep. Their Patriarchal Voices cause them to put aside their own concerns for their husbands'.

I watched a UK television documentary about young girls who deny they are pregnant. They may suppress their physical symptoms. If they feel sick they attribute it to something else. They conceal the fact they are pregnant from others and, unconsciously, also from themselves. Parents collude by accepting a negative reply when they ask their daughters if they are pregnant. Dr Meg Spinelli, psychiatrist, says these girls experience a phenomenon known as 'splitting' which causes them to separate from reality. Only when they talk about it to someone else it becomes real. Concealment, denial and splitting make it a fantasy.

The baby is born with an unassisted delivery. The girls may experience shock, horror, panic and fear. They don't howl, cry or shout. They make no noise. Dr Margaret Oates says they are like frightened animals. Still in a state of complete denial they may then kill the baby at birth, smothering it or abandoning it.

The Patriarchal Voice is probably responsible for the pregnancy in making sure the girl is compliant when approached for sex, then it keeps the girls unaware of the pregnancy and makes sure they don't let anyone else know either.

Patients

Illness is a mystery. Patients often don't know what is happening to them and doctors are often guessing. Patients give their power away to doctors.

Caroline Myss Ph.D., a medical intuitive, author of <u>Anatomy of the Spirit</u>, says illness occurs when we lose energy from one of seven energy centres (chakras) of the body. Each chakra targets a specific truth which failure to honour causes loss of energy and power. As we learn to take back power the energy loss diminishes and we heal. Sometimes we choose to remain ill or even to die rather than claim our power.

Allison's Patriarchal Voice keeps her a child and victim. She keeps the peace around her husband. She dilutes family problems and protects him from stresses and worries. Her Patriarchal Voice restricts and restrains her making her a victim. When she becomes ill she gives power to doctors, pharmacists, surgeons, anaesthetists, medical educators, physiotherapists, acupuncturists and chiropractors. She has yet to discover her own power. Her fear prevents her going within to find the emotional cause of her illnesses.

Most women are at the mercy of their Patriarchal Voices, many feel taken for granted and powerless. Some claim a form of power and get space for themselves by becoming ill. An illness is often an unconscious escape from challenges. It may be 'out of the frying pan into the fire'. These women may not know another way to overcome the difficulties they face in life.

Nurses and Doctors

Many nurses report their effort is under-valued. A trained nurse described the atmosphere in Delivery Suite whenever a nurse rang a doctor to report on a patient. "Rarely a nurse ends a phone conversation with a doctor feeling okay," she said. As an axiom nurses are under-valued by doctors. Their work and worth are trivialised and belittled. Whether a doctor is male or female many are often patriarchal.

Nurses, including midwives, are trained to give responsibility and authority of care for patients to the 'superior' knowledge and wisdom of doctors. A parent (patriarch, doctor) must have power over her/his daughter/son (nurse). Nurses are often at the mercy of their Patriarchal Voices. They react to the patriarchal energy in the doctor becoming either a good compliant daughter/son who defers to her/him or a rebellious bad daughter/son who may show her/his defiance. Either way nurses often feel like powerless children.

An example of this type of parent/child interaction is shown in the following example. A nurse phoned a doctor to report a suspected bowel obstruction in a new-born. The time was 11.30 pm. Angrily he said: "You woke me up." The angry father (doctor) chastised the naughty little girl (nurse) for misbehaving. She left the phone feeling invalidated. The system requires a nurse defers to a doctor. S/he is taught to be fearful and to take no responsibility.

If a nurse and doctor differ in opinion the nurse is at risk of becoming the victim. Senior staff rarely take the side of the nurse and s/he may be reprimanded and criticised. Often the doctor is not judged and escapes without censure. Because the Patriarchal Voice turns the nurse into a daughter/son the relationship with the doctor is already set up to be a parent/child interaction. We must become aware of this voice and separate it from our personality so that we have the power to change our relationships.

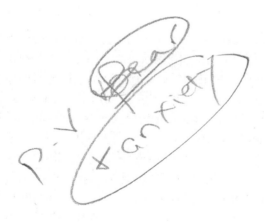

13

The Patriarchal Voice in Relationships

"What finally became clear to us was that the idea of surrender in relationship is not to another person but to the process of relationship itself."

Hal Stone Ph.D. & Sidra L. Stone Ph.D. <u>Partnering</u>

I read with fascination a book called <u>The Marriage Plan</u> by an American author. It sets out in an ordered fashion how to go about acquiring a husband within a year. It has a bright pink loose cover over a quieter variegated purple cardboard cover. The pink cover (to attract women) can be removed and a self-respecting woman can read <u>The Marriage Plan</u> secretly without feeling inadequate and embarrassed. If she can acknowledge the Patriarchal Voice, quieten its fears and settle its anxiety, she may be able to put into action the directions suggested by the book. After all the inner patriarch knows that in order to achieve a goal a plan must be followed. In order to adhere to the plan she needs to call upon the energy of the Patriarchal Voice to support an idea that it fundamentally disapproves of. It would say that a woman who does not have a partner is flawed and probably doesn't deserve one. Needless to say, this results in inner conflict.

Patriarchal society has given women the roles of wife, mother and carer and not much else. Today's woman may appreciate the freedom attained in recent years and may find she is not willing to relinquish her independence to be the traditional wife and mother.

If she marries she may feel she has settled for less. Her Patriarchal Voice can tell her she is needy and flawed because she wants a relationship. It wants her to be married and yet tells her to desire a relationship is a feminine need and therefore does not meet with approval. A woman's willingness to care, nurture, cherish and love her family members is an asset beyond monetary value. The Patriarchal Voice may not acknowledge this important priceless gift. Women's worth has been taken for granted, devalued and judged not equal to men's by the Patriarchal Voice. Women's qualities are considered less valuable compared with manly qualities.

I talked to a married friend about the Patriarchal Voice. She told me she lives in her marriage separately from her husband. He has his interests and she has hers. She discovered she had little joy if she didn't establish activities separately from her role as wife and mother. Life wasn't worth living. She is sure the marriage would have ended. This is how she coped. I suspect many marriages that survive are similar. Each partner must establish purpose and enjoyment for themselves.

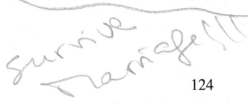

John Howard, Australian Prime Minister (the patriarch), exercised his power to silence the voices of single women when the courts granted them the chance to have a child through in-vitro fertilisation. He stepped in to quash, not just their voices but the opportunity, the choice, *the chance* to have a baby without a male partner.

Insecure men are scared to hand power to women, probably because they are afraid they will be abused by women in the same way that men have traditionally abused women. Many men believe they need to contain women. The patriarchy belittles and trivialises women and their work as a means of keeping control. In putting women down man is attempting to elevate his own position. He uses his power to keep his position as head of the system.

Men and women are different. Men can use physical force because they are stronger. Women's way of ruling and leading is different from that of men. Women are generally softer and gentler than men and they are socialised to nurture. If both men and women embrace their masculinity and their femininity we have a new way of relating. The feminine idea of both/and (holding both masculinity and femininity) offers a new perspective to the masculine duality of either/or. From the feminine viewpoint each side of a polarity completes the whole.

The ideal would be that men and women work together as equals respecting each other and valuing each other's contribution and nature. The Patriarchal Voice can be used in male and female to set boundaries and limits, handle finances, create order, make clear decisions, guard against invaders, with a wise, loving and firm hand.

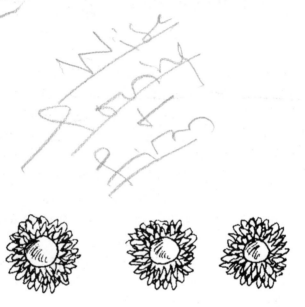

14

Disowning the Patriarchal Voice

"For most people, it takes a lifetime for the psyche to find its relationship to the Goddess. She appears in the psyche in her three-fold nature, sometimes Virgin, sometimes Mother, sometimes Crone. However it is the Crone that our culture has so brutally repressed. The wise woman, the healer, the transformer has been one of the greatest threats to the patriarchal world."

Marion Woodman <u>Dancing in the Flames</u>

In the unconscious masculine and feminine are not tied to gender. Masculine is not necessarily male and feminine is not necessarily female.

As explained by Evelynne Joffe (1996) the Hebrew myth of Lilith, demon of the night, is a myth of resentment, rejection and exile. Throughout time she has come to symbolise the patriarchy's fear of the feminine as dark and evil. The mythical figure of Lilith has been adopted by many feminist groups as an image of the feminine who refuses to be subordinate to the male. In the Jewish myth God created two lights, the sun and the moon. They were both created equal, but the moon and the sun were not at ease with each other, so God told the moon, "Go and diminish thyself." She was mortified and asked why she should "veil herself", but she obeyed Him. From that time on she had no light of her own, but only a reflected light from the sun. God said it was fitting that there were two lights, the sun to shine by day and the moon to shine by night. From the moon's resulting resentment, Lilith's energy was born.

Lilith was the original wounded feminine, not as good as a man. She is that quality in woman that refuses to be told what to do, the quality that desires freedom of choice. Lilith is the instinctual, earthy aspect of the feminine. Her sexuality is experienced as animating, hungry and natural. It is primal. She is the bitter betrayed woman. She is the part of the Goddess that has been rejected in patriarchal times - the knowledge of the dark as well as the light, the instinctual, the sexual, the acknowledgment of God the father/mother.

When we suppress or disown the Patriarchal Voice it still operates in our lives but not in a way that empowers us. This energy comes at us from a person outside ourselves who carries patriarchal energy and may treat us badly. It reacts with our own Patriarchal Voice and makes us a victim of its pronouncements.

When men and women disown the Patriarchal Voice they may attract others who carry the energy for them. They may have bosses or partners who use the energy negatively by being either inflexible, judgemental, authoritarian, harsh, lacking in feeling or lacking in respect for others - or a combination of any of these ways. The Patriarchal Voice undermines our effort, our value and our worth.

Tania has a strong Patriarchal Voice. I could feel disapproval of me when I talked to her. I felt judged and realised it was her Patriarchal Voice judging me. I felt uncomfortable talking to her. It wasn't anything I said especially. It was just who I was - my Patriarchal Voice was suppressed and was reflected back to me in Tania's judgement.

When men or women disown patriarchal energy they may lose their clarity, authority, direction, ability to lead, plan, organise, direct or take charge.

The inner patriarch is a ruler used to leading and directing. In this role he does not submit. He is powerful. He wants to be in a position of strength. If he gives his power away to others he loses himself. A disowned inner patriarch still operates in our psyche and, therefore, our lives, and we can be at the mercy of his energy and not understand what is happening. The following example may help to explain what I mean.

Recently I worked with a client called Rosalie who liked to please people. She said yes to everyone's requests. She said "Yes" to the point where she lost her Self. Rosalie was in partnership with a man who denigrated and devalued her contribution in the business. Some years ago she separated from her husband. When he became ill she took him in again. He lived with her and treated her poorly. She had disowned her Patriarchal Voice and manifested the energy in the two men closest to her - her ex-husband and her business partner. Both of these men belittled her, negated her actions and devalued what she brought to their lives. She could not understand how they could treat her so badly when she did so much for them.

After Voice Dialogue consultations, using techniques set out in the following chapter, Rosalie became aware she was responsible for allowing these men in her life and learned she had the power to change the situation. Until she separated from the energy of her Patriarchal Voice, brought it to consciousness and started to honour it in herself she could not get away from these destructive men. If she had physically removed herself from her ex-husband and business partner, without coming to terms with her Patriarchal Voice, another person carrying patriarchal energy would most assuredly take their place and she would once again be a victim. Once she recognised the Patriarchal Voice, and claimed that energy as a separate Self within, she was able to make choice about her relationships.

We need to claim patriarchal energy and use it with awareness and wisdom. It is a valuable, necessary energy we could use appropriately.

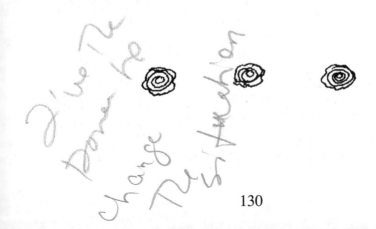

15
Voice Dialogue

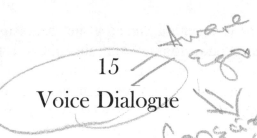

"I consider the Voice Dialogue process to be one of the most powerful tools for personal growth I've ever discovered."

Shakti Gawain in Embracing OurSelves

In the nineteen seventies Dr. Hal and Dr. Sidra Stone, American Psychotherapists and authors of Embracing OurSelves and Embracing Each Other founded a technique for talking to parts of ourselves called Voice Dialogue. The aim of Voice Dialogue is to develop a process within yourself, called the 'Aware Ego', that is able to make conscious choices based on awareness and experience of the parts that make up your personality.

Voice Dialogue is a method of talking to our inner voices. It's a way of separating them so that each can be heard individually. The therapist sits opposite the client and discovers their concern. When the client is ready the therapist asks to speak to a particular 'part' or 'voice' of the client. The client then moves away from the original seat, known as the ego position, and a sub-personality takes the new place. The therapist, inducting and holding the energy of the sub-personality, asks questions and dialogues with the 'part' or 'voice'. The client experiences the part as a separate energy and hears its comments. Awareness develops. When the client returns to the original seat an Aware Ego is beginning. Before we have an ego that is aware the dominant parts of our personality make decisions. When an Aware Ego is present we have a greater ability to make conscious choices.

Let's look at the internal dynamics of some sub-personalities. The following is a dialogue from a Voice Dialogue session with Sarah's Patriarchal Voice. After talking for a while Sarah moved her chair to one side so that the therapist could speak directly with her Patriarchal Voice.

Therapist: *I'm pleased to meet you. May I ask you some questions?*

Patriarchal Voice: *Please do. I'm keen to talk.*

T: *What is your purpose in Sarah?*

P.V: *I exist in Sarah to take care of her - to protect her. She needs protection. She's not able to do it herself. She is weak, feeble, misled, easily taken advantage of, foolish, inappropriate and a victim. I do not like her weakness. I do not like it when men take advantage of her. If she puts herself in a compromising situation and gets hurt I get furious. I am determined to protect her from now on.*

T: *You really are quite frantic, aren't you?*

P.V: *Yes, I am! I am furious! FURIOUS! She has allowed others to take advantage of her, to use her and not respect her and honour her. I do not want to let it happen again and I will do what I can to make sure it never does.*

T: *I feel your passion. Can you tell me how you developed?*

P.V: *I learned from Sarah's mother. Her mother taught me about the way things are. Women look after relationships. Their role is to make sure men are cared for, looked up to and acknowledged. Men are leaders. Women are not important. A woman must know her place and stay in it.*

T: *I see. Can you tell me how you protect Sarah?*

P.V: *She is a foolish weak woman wanting to give her power away. Men can hurt her. They have and they do. I won't let that happen to her. I'll keep her away from men. I make her look at men and not see them clearly. She doesn't see clearly. I'm affecting her thinking all the time - I look at them through her mother's eyes.*

T: *What are your thoughts?*

P.V: *My intentions are honourable. I exist to take care of Sarah, to protect her when others take advantage of her. I'm suspicious of other men. I don't trust them. I also don't like weakness.*

T: *What caused you to be this way?*

P.V: *The helplessness and hopelessness felt and often expressed by Sarah's mother affected me. I vowed not to let that happen to Sarah. I want Sarah to find out more about me and take over my job. It seems to me that Sarah does not approve of me. I'm tired and confused and mixed up. I feel lost. I need her help. I have done the best I know.*

Sarah's Patriarchal Voice is waiting for Sarah to become aware, and take over from it. If Sarah can receive the information and assess it, while also taking into consideration information supplied by her other inner voices, it can relax and not have to be the controlling energy. Now that she has become aware of her Patriarchal Voice and experienced its energy as separate from her she has the beginning of an Aware Ego. Sarah will be better able to make a choice.

Dialoguing With Your Self

Some years ago I met Lucia Cappacchione the author of several books including <u>The Power Of Your Other Hand</u>. Lucia introduced me to a way of dialoguing with parts of myself by writing with my non-dominant hand. I have used this method to heal myself regularly. I've used it to heal ailing parts of my body, illnesses, relationships and other problems that I encountered from time to time. It works!

You use Four Healing Questions to gather information. From the communication you learn what you need to do to heal yourself. Your non-dominant hand connects with your unconscious and brings to your awareness ideas and feelings you may not consciously realise.

Four Healing Questions

1. Who or what are you?

2. How are you feeling right now?

3. What caused you to feel that way?

4. How can I help you?

You can use this exercise to dialogue with your sub-personalities, with objects or people in your dreams, with people in your life, with parts of your body or with your ailments or illnesses.

You've read the dialogue of Sarah's Patriarchal Voice with a therapist. Now let's look at a dialogue I had with one of my voices that was counter to my Patriarchal Voice. I wrote questions with my dominant hand and wrote replies with my non-dominant hand. This is a marvellous exercise to find out what is causing distress and discover a solution.

Who are you?

I'm a part of you that is afraid of your Patriarchal Voice.

How are you feeling right now?

I'm lost. I've done my best. I'm now quite confused.

What caused you to feel that way?

Recent developments. I guess I'm a supporter of women and against men. I feel helpless around men. I don't like that women feel useless. I feel helpless and useless and stupid. I feel not respected and not appreciated. For example, at work I feel unappreciated.

I understand that. Anything else?

I feel strangely passive. I don't seem to do much - just react to others' ideas. My sense of self is lacking.

Why are you afraid of the Patriarchal Voice?

It talks always of men. Men first, men best. I think there could be a feeling of equality. A respect for the differences and an appreciation of them.

Do you like men?

They're about the same as women. Just people with problems and limited knowledge.

Why are you afraid of the patriarchy?

I don't like the treatment of women, the need to keep them in their place.

What personally happened to make you feel that way?

Mary was kept down in the family. Mary came second to her younger brother.

You didn't like that?

I didn't. I felt bad for her that time her father hit her and put her in the cupboard for several hours. That's when I took over. Later when she was older and he hit her I was devastated at the shocking humiliation of it all. Mary was fourteen and he pulled down her pants and hit her. I feel quite passive. Later again when Joe humiliated her I just got upset. Around strong men I lose power. I don't like the humiliation. I don't want her to suffer it.

What can I do to help you?

Mary needs protection. I can't give it. I am obviously too passive. Develop your Patriarchal Voice to protect you. You need that energy positively in your life, not as a criticism, as a protection. You are okay. I am okay. Patriarch is okay when used properly and appropriately.

From this dialogue I learned about an energy within me that felt helpless and at the mercy of the Patriarchal Voices in myself and others. This Self felt unhappy and unable to change the situation. This sub-personality was conditioned by treatment I had received at the hands of men. It was scared to stand up to men who were stronger and could hurt me. I believe many of us who have suppressed our Patriarchal Voice do so because we disapprove of some men's treatment of some women.

From this dialogue I also learned that this part that had protected me by keeping me passive was now ready for me to become aware of my Patriarchal Voice and to use it to exercise a more pro-active way to protect me, not by abusing others, but by setting limits and boundaries. Now that I was aware of these opposite parts, I was on my way to making more conscious choices.

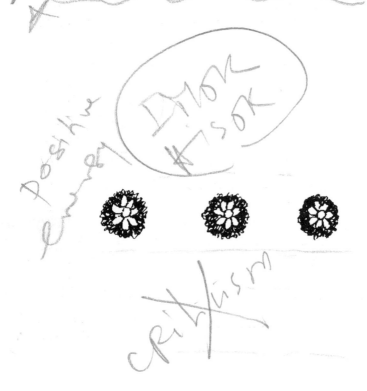

16

Protecting The Inner Child

*"If you can't get close to other people, it is because you
don't know how to be close to your own inner child."*

Louise L. Hay <u>The Power Is Within You</u>

From birth a child forms in particular ways, depending
on gender and socialisation. Studies have shown that
carers talk to a boy differently from a girl and
expectations for a boy are different from what is
expected of a girl. For example, a little girl is always
encouraged to smile. It is not mandatory for a little boy.
With changes in society the biological differences that
initially caused child-rearing to be gender based have
less impact as the need for physical strength and stamina
has waned.

In most men and women there is a natural desire for
communion with others. Many men derive a sense of
purpose in providing for and financially caring for a
family and many women in exchange offer nurturing on
an emotional level. These qualities are a function of each
individual's inner child's need for someone to take care of
them.

The inner child is a part that is always with the
individual. It is close to our essence. When we are born

we come into the world as a vulnerable child who needs nurturing and protection. As the child develops s/he takes on ways of being that help her/him to survive. These ways of being become the personality that subsequently identifies the adult.

A child may take on the energy of pleaser or pusher or responsible self or perfectionist or dreamer or patriarch, to name a few ways of being. Each of these sub-personalities, selves or energy patterns protect her/his vulnerability and assist in the child surviving to adulthood.

The inner child is protected and presumably is safe. In the process of growing up the child often becomes submerged. The personality may bury the inner child so that the 'child' aspects are lost. The inner child never really goes away but the person may have no conscious connection with the weak, playful, vulnerable part of themselves.

The inner child is a beautiful part of each person. When we 'fall in love' the child aspects come out to connect with the other person. It is a wonderful feeling to let your child out to play with the object of your affection. We let down our defences, our protective ways of being relax and stop protecting. While we are in the magic of falling in love we don't need to be defensive. Some of our (normally) hidden parts can allow themselves to be seen and we can truly feel and be with our lover's inner child. We can relax and happily let our own inner child enjoy the special moments.

'Falling in love' happens at some time to everyone. We may 'fall in love' with a new friend, house, car or job. For a while everything is wonderful. Our inner child feels loved and very safe. If only this time could last forever! Unfortunately, at some point it ends. Then the rose colour comes off our glasses and we see things in a different light.

Our usually hidden parts may go back to hiding. Our inner child goes underground. Our main energy patterns go back to being in charge of our personality and we go back to the challenges of life without the euphoria.

As a child I learned many myths and fairytales. The hero usually had to conquer challenges before he won the hand of the fair damsel who waited for rescue from her ivory tower. The hero had to fight and conquer the bull or the dragon (his natural instincts) before he claimed the fair maiden's hand. She usually just waited.

Today many women are desperate for a relationship. They tire of waiting and may venture forth before they have done the inner psychological work necessary to prepare them for partnership. They send their inner child in search of a relationship. The child is not properly cared for or protected by themselves and they are looking for someone else to nurture their inner child. A person can hurt and abandon another's vulnerable inner child intentionally or unintentionally. These women may not understand they also need to fight and defeat the bull or the dragon.

Romance novels often contain a common theme. The heroine and hero meet and clash. There is an attraction and it could be a love/hate relationship. She waits longingly while he sows wild oats and eventually comes to her. She may date another man who doesn't excite her. This one proposes marriage and she nearly accepts although she feels more chemistry with the first man. The hero and heroine usually have limited experience learning about each other's behaviours. They unite at the end of the book. He gives her a kiss that takes her 'to the moon' and they live 'happily ever after'. Many women who feel frustrated find an escape by reading romance novels. They may fantasise that this is what happens in real life.

The Patriarchal Voice keeps the female contained, restricted and waiting. She may have insufficient interests and expect fulfilment from her union with 'the one'. We must all learn to use patriarchal energy in our favour rather than be a victim to its utterances.

Embracing Your Patriarchal Voice

1. Become aware of your Patriarchal Voice.

2. Dialogue with your Patriarchal Voice. Use your dominant hand to write out questions and your non-dominant hand to write the answer. Ask the Four Healing Questions described earlier.

3. Become aware of the pronouncements of your inner

patriarch.

4. Write down the comments of your Patriarchal Voice whenever you notice them. The more you do this the more aware you will become. Also write what you hear other's Patriarchal Voices say.

5. Love yourself. This means fulfil your own needs, desires and demands. Look for the essence of the need, desire or demand and supply the essence. For example, wanting a relationship may really be needing to feel cared for. We can care for ourselves by eating good food, living somewhere we like, driving a reliable car, working in a job we enjoy with people we like and so on. If you crave companionship, first be your own friend.

Reward yourself with each step you take. Acknowledge yourself with each new awareness. When you realise you're acting in a way you no longer consciously desire give yourself a kiss or give yourself a hug with each new understanding.

6. Be grateful for everything you have, no matter how small. Count your blessings. Acknowledge what you have. The Bible states: "To s/he who has more will be added. To s/he who has not, even what s/he has will be taken away."

This is a universal generalised principle. A generalised principle is true in all cases. Mass attracts more mass.
Acknowledge what you have and you will get more.
In other words, if you acknowledge that you have

plenty of lack, you will get more lack. For example, if you complain that no-one telephones you, that will be what actually happens. Even what you have will be taken away. You will lose the things you have. The number of phone calls will diminish. No matter how few friends you have, acknowledge whom you have. Subsequently, you may be surprised to look again and see more friends.

7. Set boundaries.
Some years ago a man invited me on a date. I believed I needed to get to know a person before agreeing to have sex. I naively thought I could say "Yes" or "No" and he would accept my decision. Experience has sometimes shown otherwise. In hindsight I realise I left myself no way out. I agreed to stay the night on a boat. I was trapped and could not get away. He forced himself on me (rape). He probably believed I had given him permission by putting myself in that situation. I left in the morning at first light.

In this case my eagerness to have a relationship put me in a dangerous situation without suitable boundaries. My Patriarchal Voice was silent because my inner child was anxiously desirous of a relationship and was in charge.

Some years later I went away with a man. I discussed with him whether I was in danger of expectations of sex. He assured me I was safe, and I was. I felt apprehensive beforehand discussing the issue. It seemed silly when there had been no talk of closeness. I needed to be clear about the situation and I was relieved I was brave enough to mention it.

More recently I went away with a man and I clearly discussed the situation with him. We travelled together taking separate rooms. When he put his arm around me to initiate closer contact I reminded him of our agreement. He accepted. I was safely protected within the boundaries I had established. Our Patriarchal Voice knows how to set limits and boundaries and also knows how to be disciplined.

Financial Wealth

Many people hand responsibility for their finances to their partner and when there is a break in the relationship they may have little or no experience about financial planning.

Financial knowledge comes through experience. It isn't taught at school. It's learnt through an apprenticeship of experience and hard lessons. Once the principles are learned the Patriarchal Voice knows how to follow guidelines and how to use discipline. It knows how to save money and how to spend wisely. Its energy is valuable for applying the good money principles that enable us to invest money over time. The patriarch within can set budgets. He can create order and set guidelines. He understands discipline, rules and hard decisions. He is a leader who can protect with strength.

Both men and women can benefit from patriarchal energy. It is an archetype. Every couple needs to carry the energy. If the couple separates each partner needs to develop patriarchal energy for her/him self. In recent years society disowned this energy. The work ethic and saving and planning for the future has taken a back seat. Long term planning for retirement has been overlooked. This may explain why we are financially disadvantaged as we grow older. Anyone can become wealthy if they start saving money at a young enough age. The compounding effect of money saved with interest, and reinvested over time is one of the wonders of the world. Albert Einstein claimed it is the greatest mathematical discovery of the universe. A person on a pension can increase wealth by saving and reinvesting money over time.

These principles are not taught in school because the teachers themselves often don't understand them. They've been conditioned by financial institutions and society to spend for consumption rather than wealth.

17

Dreams

"The reason we can't see around the corner is so we don't miss the beauty here and now."

Karl Bettinger

Dreams are an excellent way to chart your progress through stages and events in your life. Writing your dreams is valuable because it allows you to read and re-read information from your unconscious. Not only that, reading your dream over is a healing practice. Your dreams are a way of releasing energy from your psyche.

Record your dreams and then interpret them to see what is happening in your life. I've recorded some of my dreams with my interpretations so you can do likewise, if you choose. Many people believe they don't dream, because their dreams escape from memory. You can get into the habit of recalling your dreams if you ask your unconscious to help you remember. Immediately upon waking write down any snippet of your dream. People in your dream represent energies in your psyche.

When I started writing I had a dream. It happened the day after an old friend reappeared in my life and said he would call me. I wondered if he would.

The dream:
There is a pathological killer locked up in a room of the house. There are three bedrooms. He has one and we have the other two. He is dangerous. Our lives are at risk continuously. I am constantly on watch. He has escaped before and done much damage. He is like Hannibal, very astute and very smart. He is ruthless and will stop at nothing to get his way. He rules us.

My heart was beating fast when I woke from this dream. I was astonished. My dream alerted me to a masculine energy that ruled my psyche. I recognised the energy of the Patriarchal Voice that had previously caused me to end relationships with men. It was ruthless and would stop at nothing. Because I was not conscious of it I was at its mercy. Until I became conscious it would continue to make sure I did not sustain a relationship with a man.

I have learned when I have a dream such as this one I am about to discover and claim an energy that has been unavailable to me.

Ten days later I have the following dream:
The baby is having its last feed from me. The child had some nourishment from both sides and then declined. I knew it was the last feed I would give her from my breasts.

This dream tells me I am becoming aware my patriarchal energy is nurtured through my feminine side. I will be protecting my inner child in new ways.

A week later I have the following dream:
The phone is ringing and ringing and ringing. In my dream I finally wake up it is ringing and I answer it. The person was just wondering what else they could do to leave a message.

This dream tells me I need to wake up and get the message.

Two days later I dream:
There are so many people staying the night I wonder where I shall sleep. One of the babies has frost-bite on her face. She is smiling still. Mum is there in a bed in a room she is sharing with many people - some of them we hardly know.

This dream tells me I am not taking excellent care of my inner child. My mother influences me in ways I do not yet know.

A recurring dream:
Someone is telling me to clear the slate and rewrite it.

This dream tells me I am able to erase some of the old patterns and establish ways of being I now choose.

Four months after the first of these dreams I dream the following:
We are getting ready to go on a long journey. There are many of us. We pack the Range Rover and get ready. I ask a friend if her parents are coming. She says no. I realise

they are too old to be interested today. I ask if I will drive. Then I decide I will drive.

For me this dream answers several questions. I learn I am willing to be in charge of my energy domain. My friend's parents represent old patriarchal energy. I realise I am moving beyond that limitation. I am equipped to go on a long journey in my life using my Patriarchal Voice through an Aware Ego. I am now ready for a new phase.

A later dream:
I'm helping at a charity that assists young people. I'm giving when I can and saying "No" too. I'm looking after the baby and giving her what she needs when she needs it. She is glad I'm hearing her and is happy because I'm answering her needs. She lets me know and I respond.

This dream tells me I'm able to hear and answer my inner child's needs. I can set boundaries.

These dreams gave me direction as I worked on transforming my Patriarchal Voice. I traced the development by interpreting my dreams. I suggest you do the same. The unconscious will bring you dreams that reflect your changes.

18
Becoming Empowered

"Life is a journey. Along the way we have experiences which give us an opportunity to learn and grow."

Mary King

Some years ago I attended a training course to be an effective presenter. I learned the importance of projecting a powerful image to make a positive statement. I decided to change my appearance. I bought new apparel and visited a hairdresser to colour my hair. In my mind I pictured a light golden brown. I settled on a shade and the hairdresser applied the cream. I waited in excited anticipation to see my new appearance. After what seemed like hours it was done. When I looked in the mirror and saw the flaming red colour of my hair I was devastated. It was a shock to see the 'new me'. The colour clashed violently with my cheeks and 'screamed' at me.

I left the salon emotionally traumatised and needing to share my feelings. I rang my mother who was busy with a visitor and had no time to talk. I quickly told her what had happened. She said: "Sue him!" That inappropriate advice did not help me.

I called my sister. She said: "Go back and tell him to do it again!" This suggestion did not help either.

My need was to have someone understand my trauma. I wanted someone to hear how I felt. I lay on my bed shaking. I was out of my 'comfort zone'. I'd spent years keeping myself in the background, inconspicuous and bland and this change meant I would be noticed and 'out there'. Finally, my daughter heard and understood.

I quickly adjusted to my new appearance. I changed my make-up to suit my hair and new acquaintances said they thought red hair was my natural colour. Changing my appearance taught me how I had restricted myself in the past (no doubt in response to my Patriarchal Voice). Staying in the background like a mouse was safer than being in the limelight attracting attention to myself. My Patriarchal Voice had kept me in the shade for most of my life. It had a tight hold on me. It kept me restricted and now I was 'breaking out'. My spirit wanted to expand and experience more of life and the transformation was well on its way.

Responsibility for our relationships begins with our relationship to our 'Selves'. If we improve our relationship with ourself our external relationships will also change for the better reflecting our internal dynamics.

When I divorced, my children went to live with their father. This loss caused me huge emotional pain. I remained open and often rang to say "Hi". I felt judged and invalidated by my ex-husband and children. It was a lonely difficult time. We were all in pain. I was at the mercy of my Patriarchal Voice and my ex-husband and children expressed theirs. I was a victim of their judgements. I puzzled why they didn't respect me. I began to realise it was because I did not respect myself. I was 'peeling the layers of the onion' getting closer to my truth. My Patriarchal Voice blamed me for the breakdown in our marriage and so did my husband and children.

Caroline Myss Ph.D., author of <u>Anatomy of the Spirit</u> says before we incarnate we make contracts with other souls. The contract may go something like the following. You and I agree that on, say, 20 September 2006, we will experience an event in which one of us will be, say, the perpetrator and the other will be, say, the victim. We agree on which of us will be the victim and which of us will be the perpetrator, and at the appointed time an event occurs with us as major players. Caroline believes a part of our purpose is to complete the contract we have already set up. If we retaliate the contract continues and a more challenging situation may arise. If we embrace and forgive the one who violated us, while also honouring and forgiving ourselves, we complete the contract. We usually don't have to repeat the experience. Although we may get a small taste of a similar situation, maybe as a test.

A business owner using patriarchal energy may not be in touch with the opposite energy. S/he may take advantage

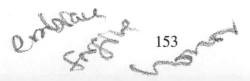

153

of employees, not appreciating their efforts, judging them and replacing them with little provocation. S/he may not be able to express her/his appreciation because this seems weak to an authoritarian business wo/man. In this situation the worker could be the victim with the boss as the perpetrator. When someone escapes this scenario forgiveness completes the contract. Retaliation continues the contract and another situation arises. Even negative thoughts toward the person who treated us badly are enough to continue the contract. Compassion, understanding and forgiveness set us free.

The goal to have an ongoing close fulfilling relationship with a man has made me continue along the path of transformation. This journey has taken time. I had much to learn and many blocks to dissolve. When a goal takes time to achieve there is something stopping us from attaining it. This could be a mental or emotional block, or it could be a belief that needs to change.

I remember some years ago I was leading a support group that met weekly at my house. After one meeting I went upstairs to shower. I was still processing an issue raised from our experiences in the group. I could 'see' in my mind a block I needed to dissipate. It was a solid block of ice as big as me. In my mind and using my arms I physically hacked at the imagined ice till it cracked open, fell away, and I broke through. I was standing in the shower holding a letter-opener that I used to symbolically hack through the ice.

Sometimes, by using an exercise like this one, we can shift blocks in our psyche. I'm sure something moved from that moment because some months later I was living in a relationship. I still had more work to do, more layers to peel, to uncover the Patriarchal Voice that was deeply embedded in my psyche. I could not sustain that relationship and it dissolved within a year.

Many of us are victims of our own Patriarchal Voice and to the patriarchs in the people around us. When we disown the Patriarchal Voice it still operates in us - judging us and causing others to judge us. It speaks to us constantly in our heads. It is a powerless position. We become victims of the people around us who use their patriarchs to limit, intimidate and devalue us. These outer patriarchs are our bosses or our partners, our mothers or our fathers, our husbands or our wives, people in our lives who rule us with an iron fist. The energy turns against us (because we are not honouring it in ourselves) and we may be treated badly by those around us.

My patriarch within protected me in the way he did because he didn't think I could look after myself. That was probably the truth. My conditioning was ingrained. He protected me by silencing my voice so I didn't upset anyone with my words, by containing me so I took up less space, by removing me from people at the first perceived injustice and by pointing out the faults in men who may have shown interest in me. He constantly reminded me of my inadequacies as a woman and of his disapproval of my efforts as a wife, mother and daughter. He didn't like mistakes. He didn't like ineffectiveness.

If we own, become aware of and separate from patriarchal energy (we can do this effectively with Voice Dialogue) we can use it as a positive force. With awareness we can use it fairly, wisely and justly. It is valuable energy.

The Patriarchal Voice can consciously set limits - as distinct from limiting us when we are unconscious of it. It uses clear thinking and can cut through waffle and red herrings. It knows when to stop, for example drinking, eating, playing, working or resting. It knows when to say: "Enough."

To be successful in the world I took on patriarchal energy. My thinking became patriarchal. I preferred talking to men rather than women. I chose the company of men ahead of women. I suppressed my emotional self and used rational thought. When I compared men and women in business, women were always a poor second. I modelled myself on men. As I was a woman I was not fully honouring my femininity and nor could I be fully masculine. I was a mimic of a man.

As I became aware of my Patriarchal Voice I realised I could be feminine and still be powerful. I discovered it is okay to bring forward more of my femininity and use it powerfully as part of who I am rather than, as before, only in ways that were approved of by the patriarchy. With each passing day I am becoming more a woman of feminine power.

The aim of this book is to bring to consciousness a potent part of women and men and to encourage the evolution of the Patriarchal Voice. Then humanity can begin partnering in this new century honouring womanhood and manhood, femininity and masculinity, supported by both the inner and outer patriarchy.

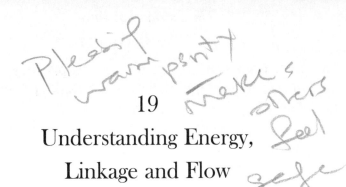

19

Understanding Energy,
Linkage and Flow

"All energy flowing in and around the body can be directed by thought."

W. Brugh Joy M.D. <u>Joy's Way</u>

When I was at school a girl in my class often used to say: "I don't care." I was impressed. I was busy caring about so many people and things I was often a victim. She didn't care. Brilliant! If we don't care we have more freedom than if we are attached. As I understand it now she was probably using impersonal energy and I was expressing personal energy. I had disowned my impersonal energy and looked in awe and wonder at her 'not caring'.

When a person suppresses or disowns the Patriarchal Voice another energy becomes dominant in the personality. For example, when I disowned my Patriarchal Voice I took on the energy of a person who is 'nice' to people, regardless of how I was treated by them. For clarity and ease of understanding we could call this energy pattern a 'Pleaser'. Pleasers care about people. They're warm and friendly in nature. Their energy field is open and extended to touch others with warmth and

159

kindness. Usually if you're nice to people they will be nice in return, your inner child will be safe. By adopting this energy pattern you protect your vulnerability. Unconsciously people feel the warmth of this personal pleasing energy.

Many women and 'Sensitive New-Age Guys' use 'Pleaser' energy. Their energy field is open and extended to touch others' fields. The dynamics of being identified with a strong energy such as the Pleaser means that because they identify with Pleaser they disown to the same (identical) extent another energy, for example the Patriarchal Voice.

Someone expressing impersonal energy expresses cooler energy. Their energy field is withdrawn. It hugs their body and doesn't reach out to touch others' energy fields. However, it isn't so retracted you feel isolated. A person sensing this energy in another feels a cooler sensation. Someone expressing the energy themselves feels cooler and clearer. The individual expressing impersonal energy is minimally affected by the other's way of being.

You may notice this energy in people serving in supermarkets or selling tickets. They impersonally serve. You don't feel abandoned (normally) but they're not personally connected to you. They really don't care about you personally. They may care impersonally - in other words they aren't unpleasant and there is an energy connection. The link is not a personal connection. Teachers often use impersonal energy. Impersonal energy gives you boundaries.

Energy in perpetual Motion

When someone is being impersonal the energy field around the body retracts. You can think with a clearer mind. You are still connected but not to the same extent. It is a cool impersonal connection. This is similar to the energy of the Patriarchal Voice. It uses impersonal energy. It can make clear decisions, set limits and boundaries, give precise directions and think sharply. When you don't have impersonal energy the effect of the Patriarchal Voice on you is extra strong.

Energy is in perpetual motion. It ebbs and flows elliptically. Where there is a void an energy will flow in to fill the space. If a person strongly carries the energy of, say, patriarch others around will express an opposite energy. It could be perhaps a sensitive, soft, more flowing energy. For example, a dominant patriarch may have as a partner a caring, pleasing person who does what s/he can to serve him unquestioningly.

In The Energetics of Voice Dialogue Principles of Transformation Robert Stamboliev describes how energy flows from one state to another. It may be full for a while and then it empties. For example when anger is expressed you may find it hard to stay angry. No matter how angry you were you can't stay that way. Once an energy has had full expression it moves away. When experiencing sadness it is hard to stay sad for a prolonged or extended period. It is when we don't express sadness, and we suppress it, say with drugs, it remains. Suppressed sadness becomes depression. By preventing its expression the emotion stays. Taking antidepressant tablets usually results in a person not having to feel depression. They may feel the need to stay on the tablets to keep the feeling suppressed.

I'm not saying don't take the tablets. Take the tablets for the present while learning new behaviours and a new inner dialogue. Unless a new way to claim the lost power is learned, it may be a life-long sentence to stay on the tablets.

In the growing-up process we take on ways of being that protect our vulnerability and control our behaviour. For example, as a baby we may see that our mother likes it when we smile. We keep smiling even when we don't feel like smiling. The repetition of this way of being that ensures we are treated well develops into a particular energy pattern we could call the 'Pleaser'.

Or perhaps instead, our parents acknowledge us for achieving. I watched a three month old baby attempting to roll over. Her parents encouraged her. She was determined to roll from her back to her front. She kept trying till finally, with a little help from mother, she rolled onto her tummy. Her carers cheered her success. They may not realise they are helping form her personality. Already she is rewarded for effort. This will probably become a behaviour pattern. She will make efforts and become an achiever. Her brother or sister born later will probably follow a different path and adopt an energy which is dissimilar, perhaps this child could be a dreamer and not be interested in achieving. Thus energy in the family balances.

Nature cannot abide a vacuum and energy flows in to fill the space. The universe is in a mathematically perfect balance of energy. If a person develops a strong energy pattern, say 'Patriarch', they will naturally suppress, repress or disown, to the same degree, an opposite energy, let us say 'Pleaser'. Someone nearby will carry Pleaser energy.

In the process of taking on an energy pattern other energies get suppressed, repressed or disowned. Again, this happens to a mathematical degree. For example we may take on patriarchal energy. Over time this can develop to a strong pattern. We may find we are always 'in charge' and we may even lose touch with how to 'play', 'allow' or 'give'. In this way the patriarchal energy causes a suppression of 'playful' or 'pleasing' energy. Later this can result in a strong patriarch drawing in a partner who only knows how to be nice and please, who may know how to 'give' beautifully but doesn't seem to be disciplined or strong. Or the partner may seem childish instead of 'sensible'. The partner may not be able to set boundaries and may be easily taken advantage of. The partner may start to feel 'used' or 'abused'.

I've seen many strong patriarchs who have partners who give generously. They are afraid to say "No". The patriarchs are frustrated and disappointed in their partners who perhaps have become like martyrs, doing everything for everybody without thought of self. Little do they know it is their own energy that causes them to draw in someone who reflects back to them parts of themselves they choose to ignore.

I say no pleasantly

We can take on a whole new understanding when we realise the people we judge are only fulfilling our disowned ways of being They reflect back to us parts of us we don't, can't, or won't express. They do this in a mathematically exact amount.

In my case I suppressed my Patriarchal Voice, as many of us do today. I drew in people I judged who also judged me. I was at the mercy of patriarchal energy in several men and women in my environment. I felt misunderstood, unappreciated and abused.

The interesting thing to know is we don't have to become like the people we judge. If I judge people for being inactive I don't have to take up smoking marijuana. All I have to do is honour the energy in me that knows how to lie back, to relax, to hang out or to 'be'. This means, firstly, I acknowledge I do have in me an energy like this, secondly, I accept it is there and thirdly I honour it. The Greeks have a good way to put this. They say we need to build a shrine to every god and goddess. The shrine need not be the same size for each god and goddess, a small shrine will do. It means acknowledging, accepting and honouring that we do have the energy we would prefer to deny as a part of our psyche. In this way we claim our shadow, the parts of our personality we have pushed out of our awareness. These sub-personalities don't lose their power in our lives because we aren't aware of them. They still affect us. They go into the world around us and return in people who carry that energy (that we can't abide) for us.

By disowning the energy we attract it in other people around us. Our partner who at first appeared ideal now seems less than perfect as we find out more about his/her ways of being and doing, things we hadn't considered at first as being a problem suddenly are bigger issues.

When we disown an energy, for example suppressing the Patriarchal Voice, it creates a vacuum. As stated before, nature cannot sustain a vacuum so it fills the void with patriarchal energy from a source outside ourselves. In other words, a person who suppresses or disowns the Patriarchal Voice draws in people around them who carry the energy and may use it to victimise them.

It is a natural phenomenon. Nature responds. That's why we need to be responsible for our own energy domain. If we suppress an energy it has to go somewhere. Usually it goes out into the world around us and draws in people who carry the energy we have repressed.

When energy comes towards us we can let it in to our energy field or we can learn to consciously keep it out. We can choose how to respond to others' energy fields. We can block energy by creating, using our mind and imagination, an invisible screen that holds the energy out.

The imaginary screen can consist of any material we choose that we believe is capable of stopping energies from encroaching on us. It could be ice (like the block I had created that prevented me from experiencing feelings) or it could be something less solid and less permanent that you choose to erect when appropriate.

By creating this screen around us we can protect our energy system. It can be raised or lowered, strengthened or made permeable, depending on what we want to let in or keep out. Energy follows thought. We create the screen in our mind and we use our imagination to make changes. Our screen could be made of glass or a flower or perspex or something more solid if we prefer. Recently I found a flower effective. By using this screen I protected myself from invasive 'negative' energy.

This method of blocking energy is able to be used when we feel our energy is being drained from us by sources outside ourself, or invaded by others whose energy we don't wish to absorb. You can wrap your energy around you. To avoid my energy being drained by others in a shopping mall, I remember being told to walk faster than the 'shopping energy'. Another time when I was doing a workshop in Bali, and felt invaded by the Balinese selling their wares, the suggestion was made to project my energy ahead to where I was going and the Balinese sellers would not approach me. That advice worked. I was able to walk unmolested.

Energy is invisible. Even though we can't see it we can feel it. It obeys the laws of the universe as if it had form.

20
Healing the Patriarchal Voice

"Learning to cherish and emphasise feminine values is the primary condition of our holding our own against the masculine principle which is mighty in a double sense - both within the psyche and without. If it attains sole mastery, it threatens that field of woman which is most peculiarly her own, the field in which she can achieve what is most real to her and what she does best - indeed, it endangers her very life."

Emma Jung <u>Animus and Anima</u>

The Patriarchal Voice has been conditioned by our families and the society we live in. It needs to be our friend. Then we can be in charge of our own lives rather than at the mercy of others. Here are some suggestions to make this voice your friend.

- Become aware of the Patriarchal Voice. This is the most important step. If we are not aware we are powerless. Become extremely sensitised to its pronouncements. Write down what you hear it say as soon as you hear it.
- Strengthen awareness by becoming finely tuned to the energy of the Patriarchal Voice in yourself and in others.

167

- Read books that increase your awareness. I recommend <u>The Shadow King</u> by Sidra Stone Ph.D. Sidra was the first to discover, bring to consciousness and name the inner patriarch. She calls him the Shadow King because he operates in the shadows of our psyche. His authority is that of a king and he rules powerfully from the darkness of the unconscious. He is too deeply embedded to be easily cast aside by the women's movement.

- Draw the patriarch with your non-dominant hand. Dialogue with him using your non-dominant hand. For more on this read <u>The Intuitive Voice</u> or <u>The Power Of Your Other Hand</u>.

- Work with your dreams, write them down, read them to yourself and analyse them. In the chapter entitled 'Dreams' I've detailed dreams I had while writing this book. By analysing your dreams you can follow the development and transformation of your Patriarchal Voice. You will find a more comprehensive guide to interpreting and working with your dreams in my book <u>The Intuitive Voice</u>.

Whether you identify with the Patriarchal Voice or you suppress or disown it, it is important to know it developed for a purpose. Depending on what life experiences happened to you, you probably used, or refrained from using the energy, for a good reason. Whatever you did, I'm sure it was necessary in your life at the time.

to protect one consciously + not to control one unconsciously

In my life there were times when I used patriarchal energy and other times when I didn't. As a woman succeeding in a man's world (especially in Australia) I used patriarchal energy. I had to. I would not have succeeded. I survived a marriage break. I ran a successful business in pharmacy for seven years. I lead personal growth workshops for four years and became a consultant for personal development. When I thought I knew the answers it was probably my Patriarchal Voice speaking (the psychological knower).

After achieving these goals I wanted to experience more of my femininity again. I decided the Patriarchal Voice had too much say and I switched to disowning patriarchal energy. Neither of these positions is ideal.

The real power lies in embracing both sides and having each available as a choice from an Aware Ego, as discussed in Chapter 15. The power comes from holding the tension of the opposites. For more on this read Hal and Sidra Stone's book Embracing OurSelves.

I now believe I am in a better position to choose, having worked with my Patriarchal Voice and coming to understand how and why I was a victim to its energy. If you follow the suggestions in this chapter you, too, can reap the rewards.

21
The Patriarchal Voice Transformed

"If we have been working to develop both sides of ourselves, we recognise that masculinity without femininity is a killer. Likewise, femininity without masculinity is a devourer."

Marion Woodman <u>The Maiden King</u>

In the twenty-first century, the age of Aquarius, outmoded forms of society will change, they will not endure. The planet Uranus, ruler of Aquarius, responsible for change in unsatisfactory, discriminatory situations, will cause changes in the social forms of expression. We see increasing numbers of men and women making public the fact that they are gay. The old patriarchal system, as it was, is being eroded and change is inevitable.

Patriarchal energy will not disappear. The energy is valuable. The ideal would be for *each of us* to embrace this energy and honour it as part of who we are. We need no longer be victims. We can bring order and clear thinking to our lives. We can live in love and not fear. If we, men and women, learn to use patriarchal energy in our own lives with consciousness relationships will transform.

A good patriarch rules with wisdom, authority, love and power. He makes decisions and sticks to them. He protects weaker members of the family. He puts things in order. He spends sensibly and wisely.

The extreme side of the patriarch, when allowed to rule without question, is that he rules with an iron fist. He discriminates against the weaker. He can be rigid with too much structure. He may be lacking in flexibility, freedom, generosity and luxuries.

We need to use the Patriarchal Voice not to attack, belittle or rape others. His value lies in being a clear leader, a cool director and a masterful organiser. He does not need to rape and pillage. His authority used in our lives with awareness and wisdom enables us to work out solutions and establish and follow directions to a goal.

Each person benefits by a balance of patriarchal energy. We have authority over ourselves. Men can be men again and women can be just as powerful in ways that value and honour their femininity. A woman can use her feminine energy safely protected by her own Patriarchal Voice. She can set her own limits and boundaries using her patriarchal energy and take charge of her own life.

The patriarch within can discriminate and he can say no. He knows when to say "enough" whether it be how much to spend, how much to play, how much to eat, how much to drink or even how much bubble bath to use! Enough is a powerful word. The Patriarchal Voice uses a sharp

I'm a Masterful Organizer

mind, the ability to decide and act on the decision putting a stop when the limit is reached.

Claim the energy of the Patriarchal Voice. Honour it and use it wisely. Use it in your life with the authority it can command, but remember to stay in charge yourself, don't let the inner patriarch dominate. Rulers can misuse their power and abuse the privilege. Sometimes you need to make tough decisions. The Patriarchal Voice is just the one to do it but make sure its decrees are appropriate.

We need to bring this energy to consciousness and use it with awareness. Others will respect who we are because they can unconsciously sense the authority of the Patriarchal Voice.

Men and women can work together as team. T. E. A. M. Together Everyone Achieves More. This idea gives value to everyone on the team. Each person makes a contribution that is appreciated as part of the team, rather than assessed separately.

Today rather than domination of women by men or other women let us have equality in partnering, men honouring their feminine and masculine selves and women similarly honouring their masculine and feminine woman energy.

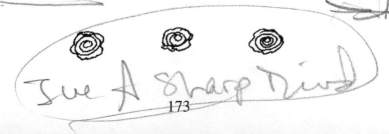

I've A Sharp Bird

A Note From The Author

If you would like to book me for a consultation please write to me at:-

**Power To Choose
PO Box 67
Hawthorn 3122
Victoria Australia**

or

Email me:-

maryking@patash.com.au

or

Visit the website:-

www.themenu.com/powertochoose

To find out more about Voice Dialogue, Trainings and other Voice Dialogue Facilitators contact:-

Voice Dialogue Australia
Phone:- **61 3 9489 9110**
Email:- **latona@ozemail.com.au**

Recommended Reading & Resources

The Shadow King
Sidra Stone Ph.D.
Nataraj Publishing
CA 1997

Business as Unusual
Anita Roddick
Harper Collins Publishers
UK 2000

The Intuitive Voice
Mary King
Brolga Publishing Pty Ltd
VIC 1999

The Whole Woman
Germaine Greer
Doubleday
UK 2000

Manhood
Steve Biddulph
Finch Publishing Pty Ltd
NSW 2000

Embracing Your Inner Critic
Dr. Hal & Dr. Sidra Stone
Harper Collins Publishers
USA 1993

The Energetics of Voice Dialogue
Robert Stamboliev
LifeRhythm Publishing
CA 1992

The Power of Your Other Hand
Lucia Cappacchione
Newcastle Publishing
CA 1988

Anatomy of the Spirit
Caroline Myss
Crown Publishers
NY 1996

Healing The Shame That Binds You
John Bradshaw
Health Communications, Inc
FA 1988

Embracing OurSelves
Dr. Hal & Dr. Sidra Stone
Nataraj Publishing
CA 1989

Bringers of the Dawn
Barbara Marciniak
Bear & Company Inc
NM 1992

Seventy-Eight Degrees of Wisdom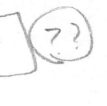
Rachel Pollack
Thorsons
UK 1997

The Maiden King
Robert Bly & Marion Woodman
Henry Holt & Company Inc.
NY 1998

Joy's Way
W. Brugh Joy M.D.
St. Martin's Press
NY 1979